Timeless

Timeless

NATURE'S FORMULA FOR HEALTH AND LONGEVITY

LOUIS COZOLINO

W. W. NORTON & COMPANY | NEW YORK · LONDON

Independent Publishers Since 1923

Important Note: *Timeless* is intended to provide general information on the subject of health and well-being; it is not a substitute for medical or psychological treatment and may not be relied upon for purposes of diagnosing or treating any illness. Please seek out the care of a professional healthcare provider if you are pregnant, nursing, or experiencing symptoms of any potentially serious condition.

For information about permission to reproduce selections from this book, write to Permissions, W. W. Norton & Company, Inc., 500 Fifth Avenue, New York, NY 10110

For information about special discounts for bulk purchases, please contact W. W. Norton Special Sales at specialsales@wwnorton.com or 800-233-4830

Manufacturing by LSC Harrisonburg
Book design by Molly Heron
Production manager: Christine Critelli

ISBN: 978-0-393-71325-1 (pbk.)

W. W. Norton & Company, Inc., 500 Fifth Avenue, New York, N.Y. 10110
www.wwnorton.com

W. W. Norton & Company Ltd., 15 Carlisle Street, London W1D 3BS

1 2 3 4 5 6 7 8 9 0

For Sam

CONTENTS

ACKNOWLEDGMENTS

I WOULD LIKE TO THANK DEBORAH MALMUD AND Andrea Costella of W. W. Norton Professional Books for their guidance, assistance, and support throughout this project. Thanks go to my friends at Pepperdine University, with a special acknowledgment to my colleagues Rachel Gradstein, Rebekka Helford, Rico Larroque, Rosalind Lee, Francesca Parker, Daniel Paraiso, Erin Santos, and Renee Sloan for their hard work, good humor, and forbearance. My respect and appreciation also go to my colleagues, friends, and wise elders Alex Caldwell, David Lechuga, Hans Miller, Cecile Schwedes, Ed Shafranske, Allan Schore, Daniel Siegel, and John Wynn—many thanks to you all.

"If we take eternity to mean not infinite temporal duration but timelessness, then eternal life belongs to those who live in the present."

—Ludwig Wittgenstein

Timeless

Introduction

It's not how old you are but how you are old.

—Jules Renard

I GREW UP BELIEVING THAT I WOULD BE AN ADULT the day I turned 18 and officially old on my 65th birthday. I suppose this is because I was told that I could drink alcohol at 18 and retire at 65. But why 65? Why not 60 or 70?

It turns out that during the 19th century, the Prussian General Otto von Bismarck was pressured to provide former military men with a pension. At first he refused, preferring to devote all of his resources to his military ambitions. Under continued pressure, Bismarck commissioned a study that found the average life span of retired soldiers to be 66 years. Armed with this information, he agreed to grant pensions at age 65, quieting his critics while controlling costs. This retirement age was adopted by industries across Europe and eventually spread to the United States. Turning 65 is but one way to think about aging. This book presents an alternative.

A RICH LIFE

I don't believe in aging. I believe in forever altering one's aspect to the sun.

Virginia Woolf

Madame Calment, the grandmother of France, died in 1997 at the age of 122. Over the years, her birthday became a citywide holiday in her hometown of Arles, with everyone turning out to honor their matriarch. Madame Calment was quite a character. From early childhood, she enjoyed playing a variety of sports, rode her bicycle for almost a century, and took up fencing at the age of 85. She personally credited drinking wine for her longevity and, despite her doctor's warnings, she consumed two pounds of chocolate a week, smoked every day, and lived to attend her doctor's funeral.

After 46 years of marriage, she and her husband Fernand had the misfortune of dining on some poorly preserved cherries. Fernand died, but Madame Calment lived on, and on—so long, in fact, that all of her immediate family and her lifelong friends passed away, leaving her to wonder if she had been "forgotten by the Good Lord." Despite her many losses, Madam Calment lived life to the fullest, enjoying people, laughter, and telling stories. She was quoted as having said, "All my life I've put olive oil on my skin and then just a puff of powder. . . . I could never wear mascara. I cried too often when I laughed." And my favorite: "I've never had but one wrinkle, and I'm sitting on it."

While accounts vary, a popular story about Madame Calment tells of a deal she made during her 90th year. A local accountant half her age, Andre-Francois Raffray, agreed to pay her 2,500 francs a month in exchange for her home upon her death. After all, how much longer could a 90-year-old woman live? With no living heirs, this reverse mortgage seemed like a wise decision for both Madam Calment and Raffray. Unfortunately for the accountant, he continued to pay her every month for 31 years until his death in 1996. To add insult to injury, his heirs continued the payments until Madam Calment's death. It is estimated that this deal netted her more than three times the value of her property.

Near the end of her life, Madame Calment, by then almost completely blinded by cataracts, was visited on her birthday by President Chirac. After being examined by the president's personal doctor, she was told that a simple surgery could restore her sight. As a gift from France, she would be taken to Paris, have the procedure, and recover for as long as she would like at the president's mansion. Without missing a beat, she replied, "Thank you, Mr. President, but no, I've seen enough." She was, according to Chirac, "a little bit the grandmother to all of us."

Madame Calment is remarkable for both her longevity and spirit, making us wonder about the possible connection between how long we live and how well we live. Her life stands in stark contrast to many common assumptions and prejudices about aging. At age 65, she had only lived half her life. As longevity increases, how will we live in the decades past 60? What will our aging be like, and how do we keep our brains active and alive? Perhaps more importantly, how do we live our lives to optimize our later years? Before we begin our exploration, let's examine some of our assumptions.

WHAT IS AGING?

How old would you be if you didn't know how old you are?

Satchel Paige

We all share the experience of material things wearing out and eventually becoming obsolete. Our cars, clothes, and furniture start out as shiny new additions to our lives but gradually become tattered, fall out of fashion, and get moved to the garage before their final journey to the trash. These everyday experiences become unconscious metaphors that shape our understanding of our physical and social worlds. Our common sense then guides us to believe that humans start out as fresh and desirable, reach their peak in young adulthood, and gradually decline into obsolescence. The more we desire the new and dispose of the old, the more this becomes the way we think of one another and eventually ourselves.

It appears to me that consumer culture and our prejudices about aging are tightly interwoven. The media bombards us with messages of how bad it is to be slow, wrinkled, and out of shape. Older adults mostly appear in advertisements for arthritis, shingles, and erectile dysfunction when not being told they need life insurance to avoid being a burden to their children. Given our present cultural values, it becomes self-evident that aging is undesirable and something to be avoided at all costs. Thus, we spend more money on plastic surgery, beauty aids, and diets than we do caring for the elders we will someday become.

Few prejudices in current Western society are more powerful than those concerning aging. And although scientists strive for objectivity, they harbor the same prejudices and biases as everyone else, searching for what they unconsciously expect to find. Because so much of what was known about the aging brain came from the study of dementia, the assumption was that the story of aging is a tale of loss and decline.

For generations, neuroscientists taught us that we are born with all the neurons we will ever possess, that critical developmental periods, once passed, were lost forever, and that "you can't teach an old dog new tricks." Because of all this, much of what I was taught in school about the aging brain was steeped in untested assumptions and out-dated ideas. These assumptions were so pervasive that only recently have scientists begun to even look at the brains of older adults who are leading active and productive lives.

Although it was known that new information could be learned throughout life, I was taught that brain develop-ment and neural plasticity were synonymous with the study of small children. In fact, positive adaptive changes in the brain were thought to cease after childhood. Fortunately, we are no longer certain about any of these "truths." For example, we know that new neurons do continue to grow in the human brain throughout life, and, as you will soon learn, the way that the brain processes information changes throughout life in line with traditional shifts in social expectations and responsibilities.

At first these revelations surprised and amazed me. But it didn't take long to realize that they made complete sense. Of course we continue to grow new neurons. Dramatic changes in our attitudes, actions, and social roles must be related to changes within the brain. As these ideas continued to fill my mind, they led to the question: What if our assumption about the adult brain as a gathering of loss was just an extension of our negative associations about aging?

THE TIMELESS SELF

> The great secret that all old people share is that you really
> haven't changed in 70 or 80 years. And that, of course,
> causes great confusion.
>
> Doris Lessing

That our brains change throughout life makes sense; that all of the changes are negative makes no sense. The simple fact that many individuals accomplish amazing things later in life defies the pessimistic dogma that has guided neuroscience for so long. What if, just like during adolescence, the brain goes through a series of modifications that prepare us for the challenges and responsibilities of each stage of life? What if the human brain progresses through a number of adaptive incarnations while our identity and sense of self remain the same?

The experience of aging is both a personal and deeply subjective experience that we seldom talk about. We complain about aches and pains and compare notes about the best doctors, but avoid exploring the landscape of our actual experience. To further complicate matters, we don't necessarily feel older. Rather, we are informed of our age by how others treat us and the heat generated by the number of candles on our birthday cake. People begin calling us ma'am and sir and offer to carry our groceries to the car. There is a point where you no longer just "look great"—you "look great *for your age*."

As a child, I remember my grandmother stopping as she passed a mirror. She would peer inquisitively at her image as if looking into an alien world. Sometimes she would press her cheeks, lift her forehead, and stare at the soft brown eyes looking back at her. "What are you doing, Nana?" I once asked. At first, she was startled by my intrusion into her private world, but eventually she began to share her thoughts. "When I go by the mirror, I expect to see one person, but instead, I see someone else," she said, "so I get scared and try to find myself. If I look long and hard enough, I can find myself, but it takes awhile. I know

I'm getting old, but I can't seem to get used to the idea that I no longer look like me."

Having no idea what she was talking about, I naively asked her who she thought she should look like. Instead of answering, she retreated to her bedroom and, after some rummaging, returned with a colorized photograph of a young girl dressed in the style of the 1920s. She had a teasing half-smile, a slight tilt of the head, and a gleam in her eyes. She handed it to me proudly and said, "This is the face I expect to see when I look in the mirror."

Now I was even more confused. Why would anyone as beautiful as my grandmother want to look like some stupid girl in weird clothes? "Why would you want to look like that girl, Nana?" I asked. "You're much prettier." She smiled and rubbed my head. "Thank you honey, but this is a picture from when I was 19. This was taken a few years before I met your grandfather, and all the boys wanted to take me dancing. For some reason, this picture got frozen in my mind. No matter how old I get, I still expect to see this girl when I look in the mirror." While her explanation made no sense to me at the time, I remember her words when I pass a mirror and find some strange old fellow looking back at me.

The fact that the experience of the self is ageless leaves us dependent upon feedback from the outer world to mark the passage of time. Like my grandmother, we must look into the mirrors available around us to reflect the passing years. These mirrors include the media, cultural beliefs, all kinds of prejudices, and our changing appearance and physical health. As with most aspects of life, our assumptions and the messages we receive influence our personal experience of aging. How wonderful it would have been for my grandmother to see herself as I saw her.

In contrast to past centuries, many of us are now looking at life expectancies well beyond 80. And while full retirement at age 65 may have been a reasonable goal of past generations, changes in longevity, economics, and culture are leading us to reconsider the meaning of being an older adult. Luckily, some of us have jobs that use our intellectual rather than our physical strength, allowing us to work longer and better than previous generations. These changes will only become greater in the future as more jobs become information based and the routine tasks of everyday life become increasingly automated. We also have the benefit of scientific discoveries that are beginning to unlock some of the secrets of aging. But if we are living and working longer, we need to take a hard look at aging, rethink what it is, and decide what we want to do with it.

It is our good fortune that the current generation reaching their 60s is not known for accepting dogma or following in the footsteps of others. As adolescents and young adults, we participated in antiwar activism, feminism, the civil rights movement, free love, and the use of mind-altering drugs. We are rethinking retirement and the role of older adults in family and society. It is up to all of us to create a new meaning of aging that will guide our culture in more positive ways in the years to come. We are well positioned to participate in a new revolution—a revolution of perspective on both aging and the brain.

MAINTAINING A HEALTHY BRAIN

We must let go of the life we have planned, so as to accept the one that is waiting for us.

Joseph Campbell

Although the focus of this book is attachment, I will begin by exploring the evolution, development, and functioning of the brain. This will serve as a foundation for a positive reframing of lifelong development in the context of relationships. We will shift from thinking about the brain as an individual biological structure trapped in one's skull to the brain as a social organ linking us to one another. From this perspective, relationships of all kinds will take center stage in the growth, regulation, and direction of each individual's biological, psychological, and social development. We will be exploring parenting, grandparenting, marriage, and other significant relationships to look at their impact on our health and longevity.

We will consider the life of the brain, the emergence of wisdom, and the implications of recent neuroscientific findings for our day-to-day lives. Through each chapter, we will shuttle back and forth between a focus on the brain and various social sciences in an attempt to grasp how each helps us to understand the other. The research on health and longevity most of us are already familiar with will be tied to the evolution of the social brain and the role our individual health plays in the survival of our relatives and our tribes. As we go along, we will find that many of the disconnected facts related to brain health make more sense when seen in the context of how the social brain evolved.

Far back into our deep history, human tribes needed elders to be responsible for preserving history, peace making in times of conflict, and nurturing the young. The older members of the tribe were sought out for practical and spiritual guidance and were in charge of the transition rituals from one stage of life to the next. We will look at the ways that the brain changes in how it processes information as we age and how these changes serve to enhance the performance of older adults in these traditional social roles. A considerable amount of time will be spent examining the nature and origins of wisdom, its role in culture, and the changes in brain functioning that make it possible. My goal is to present a unified vision of aging, grounded in relationships and expressed in lived experience—one that will increase understanding, inspire hope, and provide clues about who we are as a species and what we might do to thrive in our later years.

Part
One

BUILDING THE
SOCIAL BRAIN

1

Our Social Brains

One's life has value so long as one attributes value to the life of others.

—Simone de Beauvoir

Most scientists study individuals and their organs in isolation from one another rather than in the context of entire bodies, families, and communities. This bias has led us to think of the brain as an isolated organ and to search for technical solutions for human dilemas. Because this way of thinking has shaped our view of the natural world, it is easy to forget that we are part of a living system that we depend on to survive—from neurons to neighborhoods to nations. From conception to death, we impact and are impacted by the biology and behavior of those around us. In essence, we human beings are social animals who use our brains to connect us to one another.

Compared to other animals, humans are born with extremely immature brains and an immense number of uncommitted neurons. It is precisely this latent potential that allows our brains to be maximally influenced by the particular environment into which we are born. Thus, each of our brains is customized to fit into our unique social niche within the concentric habitats of family and community.

The layers of the fossil record of life on earth reveal the progression from single-celled organisms to increasingly complex forms of life. Over time, single-celled organisms joined together to form an amazing diversity of structures that enhanced the survival of larger organisms and groups of separate organisms. We see the progression from simple sea creatures that floated freely or attached to rocks to those that directed their own movements to search for food and mates. Eventually, sea creatures evolved into species that would come to live on land and in the air, expanding to fill the earth.

In the same way that different forms of life emerge to adapt to new environments, each species continues to evolve to better adapt to changes in the environment. In humans, natural selection favored increasing brain size as a way of expanding behavioral flexibility and eventually the development of culture. As primates evolved increasingly large brains, more brain development needed to occur after birth so that the newborn's head wouldn't be too large to pass through the birth canal and for the mother to survive giving birth. To provide for the prolonged postnatal development of less mature offspring, primates dedicated increasing amounts of energy to taking care of their young.

Groups of primates also had to develop more sophisticated means of communication and cooperation while becoming smarter about how they invested their time in hunting and gathering. Getting smarter included division of labor, strategizing, and cooperation. See Table 1.1 for a summary of those adaptations.

Table 1.1. The Interwoven Evolution of Brain and Social Structure

More Complex Brains Allow:	More Complex Social Structure Allows:
Greater adaptation	Increased role differentiation
Response flexibility	More sophisticated caretaking
Better problem solving dependency	Longer periods of childhood
Role specialization	Transmission of learning
Sophistication of attachment	The emergence of culture

In an endless cycle of reciprocal feedback and adaptation, more sophisticated brains facilitated more complex social structures, communication, and caretaking. In turn, these skills allowed for even larger brains, opening the door for the emergence of new skills and abilities.

Because our brains have evolved as social organs, they are built and regulated in the context of relationships. You know that warm feeling you get when you see an adorable baby, the reflexive wince when you see a loved one in pain, or that palpable magnetism of being drawn to someone you find attractive? These feelings, triggered by chemical processes within dedicated social neural networks, have evolved to promote bonding, attachment and cooperation, mutual care, and altruism. These everyday human experiences connect our bodies, hearts, and minds into the superorganisms we call families, tribes, and nations.

THE FABRIC OF LIFE

Our individual lives cannot, generally, be works of art
unless the social order is also.

                                      Charles Horton Cooley

Why do humans have such complex social relationships? Is all the gossip, drama, and social ritual really necessary? Mother Nature certainly loves to combine simple structures to create more complex forms of life.[1] Bacteria, ants, and gazelles have all evolved as interdependent systems. The behaviors of colonies, armies, and herds provide a level of adaptation beyond that of individuals. Penguins stand together in large groups during cold weather—the ones on the outer edge burrow toward the center for warmth while those toward the center, who are warmer, relax and drift to the colder periphery. In this way, a group of a certain size can survive as a whole in an environment where a smaller group or an individual could not.

If we assume that the social brain has been shaped by natural selection because complex relationships enhance our chances of survival, more sophisticated social groups not only allow for but require larger brains. That in turn allows a greater variety of adaptive responses in and across diverse environments.[2] Bonding, attachment, and caretaking provide the necessary scaffolding for the prolonged development required to build larger brains.[3]

Focusing for a moment on the inner workings of the brain, we discover countless neurons combining to form neural networks dedicated to specific functions such as smell and memory. These networks connect with one another, creating the capacity for even more complex abilities, such as remembering the smell of your grandmother's cooking or your grandfather's corny jokes that made everyone groan. This process plays out in a dramatic way early in life as children first develop visual abilities and motor skills and later combine them to perform more complex visual-motor skills, such as playing catch.

At a microscopic level, we find that individual neurons are separated by small gaps called synapses. These synapses are inhabited by a variety of chemical substances that allow neurons to communicate with one another. Instead of words or symbols, neurons use tiny packets of neurochemicals that allow them to connect and be sculpted into the functional neural systems that we just discussed. Over vast expanses of evolutionary time, the brain's ability to build complex systems has grown ever greater to meet our needs for increasing complexity.

When it comes down to it, doesn't all communication between people, as complex as it is, consist of the same basic building blocks? When we smile, wave, say hello, and hug each other, these behaviors are sent through the space between us via sights, sounds, and touch. These messages are received by our senses and converted into electrochemical signals that quickly travel to our brains. Our brains then respond to these signals and generate messages that we send back across what could be called a social synapse to reach others. As a result of our relationships, millions of changes within and between neurons combine and organize to shape our emotions, our personalities, and the experiences of our day-to-day lives. Through interacting with others, we activate our senses, regulate our brains and bodies, and change the shape of our neuronal structures. We build the brains of our children through our interactions with them, and we keep our own brains growing and changing throughout life by staying connected to others.

Imagine a grandfather putting his grandson to bed, and think about what is being transmitted across the social synapse. They might talk about the day and read a story while lying next to each other. As they read the story together, they share excitement, talk about the characters, and interpret its lesson. They share smells and sounds; the grandfather might move the child's hair out of his eyes, kiss his cheek, and at the end of the story, say, "I love you, honey." Positive interactions such as these likely result in increased metabolic activity and neural growth in both of their brains. Their relationship results in a new being—grandson-grandpa—and an internal biological environment in both of them supportive of secure attachment, neural plasticity, and sustained health.

However, as much as we focus on and learn from these internal biological processes, we have to keep in mind that neurons are embedded within our brains, our brains are embedded within our bodies, and our bodies are embedded within relationships. Nature repeats her strategy of combining neurons into functional systems when she combines individuals into families and tribes. In this way, there is a direct connection between what happens within our bodies and in our relationships with those around us. This is why people are healthier and live longer if they are engaged in a greater number of positive relationships. It is also important to remember that, although all people are linked together, cooperation and interdependence can be a challenge.

COMPETITION AND LOVE

All the people like us are We, and everyone else is They.

Rudyard Kipling

One of my earliest childhood memories is of a scene from an old black-and-white movie. Burned into my mind is the image of an Eskimo family traveling across the tundra in a snowstorm. The children, packed deeply into a sled, are followed on foot by their parents and their maternal grandmother. It is bitter cold, and the wind-driven snow cuts their faces as they push forward.

As the camera pans out, it becomes obvious that the grandmother is lagging behind as the gap between her and her family gradually increases. As the camera continues to pan out, we see a pack of wolves following strategically at a distance. The old woman eventually stops in her tracks, and her children, sensing her absence, stop to look back at her. Pan in close to their faces. Her expression lets them know she is ready to stay behind, and after the family's brief gesture of goodbye, the sled moves on. Pan out wide. The old woman is motionless as the sled shrinks in the distance and the wolves cautiously approach.

I was horrified! How could her family leave her behind? I ran to tell my grandmother. She listened closely as I breathlessly told her every detail I could remember. When I was done, she tried to explain to me that some families don't have the luxury of taking care of old people. "Life was very hard for the Eskimos. There wasn't much food, and children must always come first. That's the law of nature." I didn't find her words the least bit comforting. Agitated and upset, I told her that I would never leave her behind in the snow for the wolves to eat. "But the wolves have to eat too," she told me. "Let them eat cheese!" I said as I stomped away. "I hate that stupid movie." As an adult, I understand what she was trying to teach me, but I still don't like it.

Respect for the aged based on their experience and longevity has been found to be essentially universal in primitive cultures.[4] This reverence continued into the early history of Western civilizations and in the formation of Rome and Sparta. The Senate of Rome (from the Latin *senex*, meaning aged) and the Gerusia of Sparta (from *gera*, meaning old) reflect the carryover of the tribal authority of elders into the origins of the first Western governments.[5] But despite the traditional authority of age, the generations are also in competition for resources, respect, and power.

As my grandmother hinted, even if the elderly are revered, they are expected to contribute to the group. When they are no longer able, due to mental or physical disability, they become a burden, and attachments become strained. In some cultures, abject dependency is a stage of life considered to be "beyond elder," when people are thought to be overaged, dying, or already dead.[6] In some tribes these people are encouraged to commit suicide, participate in rituals during which they will be killed, or are abandoned by the tribe to the elements. Are these ancient customs precursors of our present strategy of warehousing the elderly in nursing homes?

Over the last two centuries, economic, demographic, and cultural shifts in Western society have greatly altered the relationship between generations. Prior to the invention of retirement, most people worked until they died. During the early 1800s, life expectancy in the United States was around 60 years. Life was hard, and most people expended all of their energies in day-to-day survival. Over the next century and a half, cultural changes had a huge impact on both longevity and lifestyle. By 1950, life expectancy had increased by 10 years, most children were out of the family home while parents were still in their 40s, and planning for retirement became a normal aspect of middle-class life.

During this period, the shift from an agrarian to an industrial society tilted the balance of wealth and power to a small group of elders. In agrarian societies, the family resources are tied up in land, buildings, and equipment that are shared by all generations. In industrialized societies, resources are possessed by individuals and can be used by older adults for their exclusive purposes. After a few generations of industrial growth, a relatively small group of elders in America grew to hold a disproportionate amount of the wealth. This trend has continued today via the banking, real estate, and technology industries.

On the other side of this shifting economy are a vast number of older adults who depend on benefits paid for by the working young. As we all know, the present system of Social Security in the United States is growing less viable. In 1945 there were 42 workers to contribute to the benefits of each retiree. By 1965, the number of workers was down to four, and by the year 2000, down to three.[7] Only so much of this disparity can be made up for by increasing productivity. The potential longevity and dependency of a large portion of today's older generation will, of necessity, impact the relationship between the generations. This is, of course, if older adults are as dependent as they are thought to be. As we will see later, new research suggests that older

adults contribute more and require less than we have been
led to believe.

THE EVOLUTION OF COOPERATION

*Great discoveries and improvement invariably involve the
cooperation of many minds.*

Alexander Graham Bell

As we look back through time to discover our cultural origins, human voices soon fall silent. Beyond the few thousand years since the appearance of the written word, the
only direct evidence we have of human culture are the bones
and artifacts of our distant ancestors. We add to our knowledge by comparing our brains to those of other species and
our behaviors and rituals to those of other cultures.

My first contact with the notion of evolution came during elementary school field trips to the natural history
museum, which always included a visit to the "caveman"
exhibit. We filed past life-size dioramas depicting scenes
of hunting, tool making, and cooking in a series of musty,
mahogany-paneled rooms. Some of the cavemen were eating
leaves and grinding grain into meal, while others were building fires and sharpening rocks into tools and weapons. We
were told that as humans got smarter, they were able to kill
and cook bigger animals, consume more protein, and grow
larger brains. These brains allowed them to invent more
sophisticated weapons and become more efficient killers.

The survival of the fittest seemed to mean that those who could run the fastest, jump the highest, and build the most deadly weapons would be the ones to survive.

It turned out that this interpretation of the survival of the fittest had everything to do with the propaganda of the Cold War but little to do with evolutionary theory. For Darwin, fitness wasn't a matter of physical fitness, but the goodness of fit between an animal and its environment. Each niche has factors, such as food availability, temperature, and water supply, to which living things need to adapt in order to survive. Natural selection directs the course of genetic evolution over generations through the survival and repro-duction of those who are the best fitted for the demands of each particular environment. So while you and I may be a good fit for the suburbs of Cleveland, we would be a bad fit for living underwater or on the Arctic tundra. For those environments, an octopus or penguin are fitter than we are, no matter how many push-ups we can do.

Another important bias in these dioramas was that survival was depicted as depending on the strength of the men and not the sophisticated caretaking capabilities of the women. Women were depicted as being almost incidental to the expanding brain size of the ever stronger and smarter men. In fact, it was the evolution of the social brains of the women that allowed for the sophisticated care of the ever less mature children they were giving birth to. Where would these brave male hunters be without them? It is the com-plexity of the group and the differentiation of the male and

female brains that allowed for the level of adaptational flexibility that human groups attained. Obviously, ageism isn't
the only prejudice that guides scientific theory.

For humans, our brains are our most important survival
tool, and relationships are our primary niche. This is why
emotional nurturance, attachment, and specialized caretaking are central to the evolution of the social brain. Without dedicated and emotionally attuned caretaking, there
would be no tool making, abstract reasoning, or culture.
And improving the quality of life at this point in our evolution requires that humans are able to recognize and embrace
the primacy of attachment, compassion, and wisdom. These
have always been central to the way that elders contribute
to tribes.

Consistent with what has likely gone on for untold generations, it has been estimated that over 14 million seniors
provide care and attention for their children and grandchildren in the United States. At an average of 13.7 hours each
week, their annual contribution to the social economy has
been estimated to be somewhere between $17 billion and $29
billion.[8] This contribution, often unaccounted for and taken
for granted because no money changes hands, would be difficult to impossible for many families to replace with hired
help. This was certainly true in my family. After getting
married in her early 20s, my paternal grandmother never
again brought home a paycheck. Yet she nurtured us and
served as a model of love and caring for her children, grandchildren, and great-grandchildren. She was central to the

social economy of our family and our monetary economy by keeping the rest of us going.

As men grow older, they often become more nurturing, softer, and dare I say, more feminine. Growing up, it was my grandfather who had the time and patience to answer my endless questions, let me win hundreds of games of checkers, and tell me stories of his youth. My father, then in his mid-20s, was busy building a career and forging his identity. My father and grandfather didn't always see eye-to-eye; my grandfather tried to get my father to follow his advice while my father exerted his independence. My grandfather and I, free from father-son tensions and expectations, adored each other and formed a strong alliance. It has been said that the reason grandparents get along so well with their grandchildren is because they share a common enemy—the middle generation. There may be some truth to this.

The fact that my grandfather lived well past child-rearing age gave me a crack at being fathered in a way that my own father could not provide. Those countless hours are still inside of me and help me to feel valuable and to nurture others. Those hours were an investment in the social economy of our family, part of the reason I stayed in school, and how I was able to cope with the stress and strain of daily life. Many years later, I volunteered to be a Big Brother and was paired with an 8-year-old boy to whom I gave the same kind of consistent care and attention that my grandfather gave to me. I sat with him, answered thousands of questions, and simply gave him

my time. We are still in touch 50 years later, and he tells me ...
feels many of the same things for me that I feel for my grandfather. Now with my son, I often feel my grandfather inside me
as I pass on the gift of time, affection, and love to him.
Our increased longevity, hard-won wisdom, and deeper
self-awareness are resources we can invest in others. A new
conception of aging that incorporates these traditional, non-
economic contributions to the family requires revised myths,
new heroes and heroines, and stories of wise and compassionate elders who are available, loving, and nurturing. Let me suggest a vision of the wise elder as a resource who possesses
emotional intelligence, is securely attached, and deeply enjoys
connecting with others—in essence, the embodiment of what
we all need from others to grow physically, psychologically,
and spiritually strong. A wonderful gift of evolution is that
an ongoing investment in nurturing other human beings is
also an investment in our own health and longevity. Thus, a
sustained contribution to our tribe is part gift, part obligation,
and part self-interest. Perhaps looking back at an old myth will
help to inform the new story of aging we need to create.

THE THREE SISTERS

Alone we can do little. Together we can do so much.

Helen Keller

While Western society promotes the perfection and independence of the individual as their highest accomplishment,

primitive tribes were mainly concerned with the interdependence of their members. It is clear to those who live in subsistence cultures that survival is a team sport. We find an example of this in the creation myth of the Iroquois where corn, squash, and beans are referred to as the three sisters. The three sisters provided the Iroquois the carbohydrates, protein, and vitamins they needed for survival.

In late spring, we plant the corn and beans and squash. They're not just plants —we call them the three sisters. We plant them together, three kinds of seeds in one hole. They want to be together with each other, just as we Indians want to be together with each other. So long as the three sisters are with us we know we will never starve. The Creator sends them to us each year. We celebrate them now. We thank Him for the gift he gives us today and every day.[9]

The three sisters represent a common form of companion planting—a farming strategy that places plants in proximity for mutual benefit. The corn grows straight and tall, providing a solid structure on which bean vines can grow, as well as shade and protection from pests that attack its two sisters. With its broad leaves and chemical secretions, squash conserves water, provides ground cover, and controls weeds. Beans have prickly vines that deter animals and, through a symbiotic relationship with rhizobium bacteria, take nitrogen from the air and convert it to a nutrient on which the corn thrives. Together, the three sisters enrich one another and prepare the soil in ways that enhance next year's planting.

Like the three sisters, the three human generations of an extended family have traditionally been interdependent and mutually supportive. In countless ways, the presence of each generation helps the other two. But just as the development of industrial farming led us to forget natural methods of companion planting, the value of intergenerational companionship has faded from many of the nuclear families in our modern world. Children provide the family with meaning, a shared focus, and a connection with the future. Parents support the family through childbearing, parenting, and hard work. Grandparents contribute their time, work, wisdom, and provide attachment, bonding, and support to their children and grandchildren. Like the three sisters, each generation stimulates the brains of the other two in ways that promote health and emotional well-being.

We have gone though a century when advances in culture, technology, and communication have overshadowed basic human experience. At the beginning of the 21st century, we are once again discovering the importance of attachment, self-awareness, family, and community. We have to ask ourselves: Do we cherish and celebrate our elders like Madame Calment, or do we leave them to the wolves? Do we encourage relationships between our parents and children, or do we isolate the generations for the sake of efficiency and convenience?

The generations need to interact with one another, not just for pleasure but for mutual nourishment that will help them both to grow and flourish as social beings. Young people need to be reminded that they will one day be old, just as older people need to be reminded of the child that still lives within them. As we will see, considerable evidence supports the theory that secure attachment and sustained relationships result in both better early development and healthy aging. The fundamental need to connect, interact, and love is as powerful at 100 as it is at birth.

LOVE AND LONGEVITY

Age does not protect you from love, but love, to some extent, protects you from age.

Jeanne Moreau

I'm sure you have seen hundreds of books promising the secrets of how to stay young. Most of these books are written by epidemiologists who explore the behaviors, biologies, and lifestyles of large groups of people. Based on their work, we have learned people who don't drink and smoke live longer, and those who do crossword puzzles and engage in stimulating and challenging professions are less likely to lose their memories. Exercise and fish oil, good; sloth and French fries, bad.

An epidemiologist with a slightly different twist is David Snowdon.[10] In his book *Aging With Grace*, he describes his long-term study with the School Sisters of Notre Dame, a group of nuns who came to Snowdon's attention because of their unusual longevity and low incidence of dementia. His aim was to discover the relationships between the sisters' sustained brain health and factors such as intelligence, diet, and exposure to environmental toxins. The sisters were of special interest to him because of the homogeneity of their environment and the wealth of historical information available about them.

Hundreds of nuns agreed to participate in Dr. Snowdon's study, and the majority agreed to bequeath their brains to him for anatomical analysis upon their deaths. Like most epidemiologists, Snowdon searches among biochemical, environmental, and lifestyle correlates to better understand the causes of diseases, in this case, dementia. As Snowdon began to analyze his data, he found that healthy longevity correlated with having obtained a college degree. While this finding was not new, it was of special interest with the sisters. In the general population, not having a college degree also correlates with smoking, substandard housing, less health care, and lower socioeconomic status, making it difficult to tease out if the lack of a degree is, in itself, meaningful. With the sisters, however, all of these factors were controlled for by their common lifestyle and general lack of vices. The lives of the sisters suggested that something related to having a college degree may be directly related to sustained brain functioning later in life.

Still on file were the personal statements written by these nuns as part of their initial vows five or more decades earlier. When Snowdon examined these essays, he found that those with richer vocabularies in late adolescence and early adulthood were less likely to develop dementia. This finding led to an analysis of the complexity and depth of the content of these essays, both of which were found to be related to higher cognitive functioning later in life. These findings suggest that dementia may not begin in late adulthood, but may be a lifelong process that begins in childhood or adolescence.

An alternative explanation is that people who start off bright and approach life as an ongoing learning experience continue to build new neural structures that cushion them from the effects of dementia. That is, stimulating and challenging your brain from early in life allows your brain to be more resistant to dementia and other diseases. Upon further analysis, Snowdon also found that a correlation existed between longevity and emotional expression in the nuns' essays as young women. This led him to suggest that intelligence and the capacity to articulate your emotions may both have a relationship to sustained brain health.

I smiled often while reading *Aging With Grace* because of the way Snowdon wrapped his scientific findings in a love letter to his research subjects. He clearly cared a great deal for them, and the feelings appeared to be mutual. He described the nuns as having become part of his extended family, while he became like a favorite nephew, receiving gifts of hand-knitted mittens and being included in their prayers. As I read further, the deeper meaning of his research began to emerge. The connections the nuns have with one another and even with the young researcher are part of the story. The respect, consideration, and caring they showed to one another may be powerful medicine. I began to think to myself, "Measure caring! Measure love!"

Snowdon grew closer and closer to the treasure and, by the end of the book, he transcended the boundaries of his scientific training. Describing his observations of the nuns' shared meals, he says:

> What I know for sure is that nutrition for healthy aging is not just about eating certain foods or downing a certain number of milligrams of a prescribed number of vitamins each day. It also depends on where we eat, whom we eat with, and whether the meal nourishes our heart, mind, and soul as well as our body.[11]

From my perspective, *Aging With Grace* is a story of how the interweaving of the sisters into a lifelong extended family influenced their health, brain functioning, and longevity. I believe that all members of the community, healthy and ill, benefited by their interactions and commitment to one another. We might go further to speculate about the effects of Dr. Snowdon's relationships with the nuns on his future health and longevity. I doubt he left unaffected by their caring and warmth.

ONE LOVE

You must be the change you wish to see in the world.

Mahatma Gandhi

Although searching for the connections between health and longevity is important, there is a deep and abiding story beneath the statistics. The key to the story is that the brain is a social organ that evolved to survive and thrive while interwoven with other brains. We will explore this deeper story—the life of the social brain—from the perspective of interpersonal neurobiology. Interpersonal neurobiology is grounded in the recognition that humans are best understood when studied in relationship to one another. This relatively new field emerged from an interest in the application of neuroscience to our experiences as parents, therapists, and teachers.

From birth until death, each of us needs others to care for us, help us to feel safe, and give us a reason to live. Regardless of age, relationships join people together in interactions that stimulate, build, and change the brain. In examining these lifelong processes, we will utilize findings from the neurosciences, evolutionary theory, cross-cultural studies, and developmental psychology. Through this exploration we seek to discover the workings of experience-dependent plasticity, or the ways in which the brain is constructed, regulated, and changed by our experiences with others and the world around us. We will explore how relationships impact our brains, which kinds of relationships foster brain health, how relationships make us happier and healthier, and how the brain responds to changing social demands.

The vital link between interpersonal experience and biological processes within the brain makes us particularly interested in the impact of relationships throughout the life span. The nurturance we receive from early caregivers can set us on a course of physical and psychological health, just as interactions throughout life are a primary source of brain regulation, growth, and healing. Friendships, marriage, psychotherapy, parenting, grandparenting—in fact, any meaningful relationship at any time of life—can activate neuroplastic processes, changing the structure and function of the brain.

Put in a slightly different way, human brains depend on connection and communication to survive and thrive. Stimulation, challenge, and being needed by others tell the brain to be alert, learn new things, and stay in shape. Lack of stimulation, repetitive routines, and isolation tell the brain to direct the body's energy elsewhere. While many of us work hard to earn the right to be comfortable and avoid challenge in later adulthood, this strategy runs the risk of sending our brains the message that they no longer need to grow. From a neuroscientific perspective, this is probably the worst message you can give to your brain. Fortunately for us, our children and their children need us to help build their brains, hearts, and minds. Our continued participation in the cycle of life and our ongoing contribution to the social economy are exactly what we need to maximize the quality of our own lives.

Based on these premises, I believe that a core component of ongoing health and longevity lies in the power of sustained intimacy, attachment, and learning. It is the power of being with others and staying engaged in taking on the challenges of life that builds, shapes, and sustains our brains. The best overall environment for a healthy brain is one that optimizes challenge and maximizes attachments. Therefore, how we think about aging, maintain our relationships, and stay connected to others are all vital aspects of our continued health and longevity.

2

Connecting to Others

Now join your hands, and with your hands
your hearts.

— William Shakespeare

Now that we've explored the evolution of the social brain and our interconnection with others—from caretakers to family, tribes, and community—we turn our focus to the ways we attach and stay connected. As social animals, our brains are built through reciprocal interactions across the social synapse. Being a member of a complex society requires a brain equipped to process a vast amount of social information and adapt to a changing constellation of relationships. Nurturing, caretaking, and playing all trigger a symphony of processes that promote health and well-being. For humans, relationships are our most important habitat.

We begin life with the task of getting to know those around us. This is why newborns come equipped with an array of reflexes designed to help them bond, attach, and communicate their needs. These reflexes (such as grasping, crying, and smiling) trigger caretaking instincts in parents that start the dance of attachment. During the early months and years of life, the neural circuits of the social brain are built through experience. This means that the chemistry and anatomy of the brain are shaped by the child's interaction with caretakers. These networks remain adaptable throughout life and are the same structures that adults rely on to nurture one another, be good parents and grandparents, and make new friends later in life.

From the first moments of life, we learn about the world through the attention and care we receive. The availability and quality of early caretaking shape our brains, and with sufficient nurturance, attention, and care, set us on a course for psychological and physical health. As we grow, our brains convert these experiences into biological processes that influence the ways in which we relate to others, the feelings we have about ourselves, and our implicit expectations for the future. How we bond and stay attached to others is at the core of our resilience, self-esteem, and physical health.

ATTACHMENT

Love is an irresistible desire to be irresistibly desired.
                                                    Robert Frost

Attachment is a general term used to describe the physical and emotional connections that link us to one another. And although attachments to our children, spouse, family, and friends are all somewhat different, they depend upon common biological processes that make us feel good when we are together and anxious or lonely when we are apart. Although usually studied in the context of parent-child relationships, an array of attachments are important for all of us throughout life. When a woman holds her great-grandchild, each is stimulating the other's brain to release chemicals that enhance well-being, support neural growth, and improve immunological functioning. Similar biological processes can become activated among members of a combat troop, a church choir, a sports team, or a study group. Attachments in all forms have their evolutionary roots in the bond between mother and child.

Attention to human attachment began with the psychoanalyst John Bowlby, who first noticed the similarities of interaction among humans and primate mother-child pairs. It became clear to him that primate children thrive under the care of attentive, loving, consistently available adults. As he observed the delicate balance between physical contact and exploration, he developed the concept of the parent as a *secure base* for a child's exploration of the world. Bowlby also noted that when children become stressed or uncertain, they engage in *proximity seeking* by returning to their parent until they once again feel safe to explore again. And finally, he believed that early caretaking experiences resulted in an *attachment schema*, which is the child's unconscious expectations of others' abilities to make him or her feel safe.

Bowlby's observations and ideas were taken up by generations of researchers who studied attachment through in-home observations and experiments with mothers and children. Attachment schemas in young children are measured by observing children's reactions to stressful situations and how they use their parents to regulate their fear and anxiety. Under stress, securely attached children go to their parents, interact with them for a while, and then resume exploration and play. Insecurely attached children become overly clingy, avoid their parents completely, or even engage in odd behaviors such as spinning, hitting their heads, or falling to the ground. Bowlby's work and the research he inspired uncovered connections between early attachment experiences and well-being in adulthood. It also demonstrated the importance of consistent caretakers and physical contact for children in hospitals and orphanages.[1]

Attachment schema are thought to be unconscious memories of our experiences in early relationships that stay with us for the rest of our lives. They impact our development, the quality of our relationships, and our ability to regulate our emotions. Securely attached children seem to internalize their parents as sources of inner comfort.[2] The resulting states of mind, brain, and body serve as a secure emotional base from which to establish future positive relationships.

LOVE BECOMES FLESH

*The meeting of two personalities is like contact of two
chemical substances: If there is any reaction, both are
transformed.*

Carl Jung

In recent years, Bowlby's conception of attachment has
crossed over into the biological sciences. Research has
focused on the influence of interpersonal experience on the
shaping of neurological structures and biological processes
involved in emotional regulation, learning, and bodily
health.[3] The emerging field of *epigenetics*, which studies
how experience influences genetic expression, is giving us
new tools to understand how love becomes flesh. Particular
attachment behaviors have been found to parallel structural and metabolic processes that can be measured in levels of neurochemicals, neural connectivity, and patterns of
brain activation.

The structures and regulation of these systems become
established early in life and organize enduring patterns of
arousal, reactivity to stress, and interpersonal behavior.
Secure attachments have been found to build the brain
in ways that optimize emotional regulation, learning, and
resilience. Insecure attachment builds brains that are vulnerable to stress, makes learning more difficult, and correlates with poor coping abilities. Fortunately, ongoing neural
plasticity throughout life allows us opportunities to alter

these networks by engaging in positive relationships with caring others.

We now have a biological as well as psychological understanding of why those of us who grow up in a safe and loving environment tend to be happier and healthier adults. The psychological explanation is that early relationships teach us that we are valuable and loved and that the world is a safe place. The biological explanation lies in the construction and regulation of multiple social and emotional brain systems that support resilience.

But what are these structures and systems and how do parents and grandparents support their development via nurturing relationships? A number of brain systems have been identified as being experience dependent; that is, they require positive human interactions for optimal development. Table 2.1 contains a list of some of the neural networks and biological systems that are shaped by early caretaking experiences.

Table 2.1. Experience-Dependent Social Brain Systems

Attachment System: Orbitomedial prefrontal cortex, amygdala, cingulate, insula, spindle cells, and mirror neurons

Social Engagement System: Development of the "smart vagus," which fine tuned our level of arousal to match situations

Social Motivation System: Development of social reinforcement and regulation via oxytocin, testosterone, vasopressin, and dopamine

Stress Regulation System: Benzodiazepine and endorphin receptors in the amygdala and locus coeruleus and cortisol receptors in the hippocampus

Although our understanding of these processes is still at an early stage, we are beginning to get a sense of how the sculpting of these brain systems during early experiences influences our functioning throughout life. By extension, it is through the ongoing stimulation of these circuits that we stay healthy, vibrant, and alive. Let's take a brief look at a few of the most important social brain systems. As you read through them, keep in mind that they are both interwoven and interdependent on one another. If you find that you would like to explore the social brain in more depth, please refer to my book *The Neuroscience of Human Relationships*.[4]

The Attachment System

An important component of our social brains is a portion of the prefrontal cortex that lies above and between our eyes called the orbital-medial prefrontal cortex (OMPFC). This is the first region of the prefrontal lobe to develop during childhood because learning how to connect to those around us is our first order of business.

Richly connected with core networks of learning, memory, and emotion, the OMPFC organizes our attachment schemas, emotional regulation, and ability to cope with stress.[4] These networks are built during childhood via physical contact and emotional attunement between parent and child, facilitating our lifelong connection with others.

Although we usually think of the cortex as directing our thinking and behavior, one of its primary jobs is to inhibit and regulate more primitive, basic impulses and emotions. The OMPFC plays this kind of regulatory role with the amygdala. The amygdala is in charge of activating our fear response and is fully developed by about 8 months of pregnancy. The OMPFC allows us to learn to be soothed by others early in life and later by our own thoughts, memories, and behaviors. The attachment behaviors described by Bowlby reflect the OMPFC's ability to modulate fear activation in the amygdala. One way to think of secure attachment is that the OMPFC has successfully learned to modulate the amygdala.

The cingulate cortex, contiguous to the OMPFC, evolved in mammals with the appearance of maternal behavior, nursing, social communication, and play. The cingulate cortex also contains spindle cells, which connect diverse areas of the brain that are involved in bonding and self-awareness.[6] Adjacent to both the OMPFC and the anterior cingulate, the insular cortex is involved in the integration of cognitive and emotional processing and mediates emotions, from pain to disgust to love.[7] Both the cingulate and insula become activated when we, or those we love, experience physical pain and other emotions. The degree of activation of the cingulate and insular cortexes have been shown to correlate with our awareness of our inner emotional states as well as the amount of attunement and empathy we experience with others.[8] The same neural networks involved in connecting with others also serve our ability to connect to ourselves.

Central Attachment Circuit

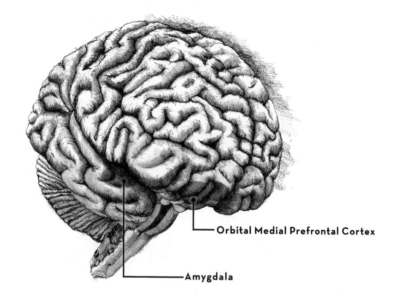

Orbital Medial Prefrontal Cortex

Amygdala

Our best guess is that attachment schemas reflect the learning histories that shape the interconnections among all of these structures, especially the OMPFC and the amygdala. These cortical structures give input to, guide, and regulate the amygdala's level of activation in different situations; in other words, when we should experience fear. At their core, attachment schemas reflect our ability to use our proximity to others to regulate fear and anxiety.

Mirror neurons also play an important role in attachment by automatically connecting our actions to those of others through imitation and creating internal models of others' experiences. Have you ever started to laugh because you found someone else's laugh infectious? How about looking up or yawning because others were doing so? These are examples of mirror neurons at work. Mirror neurons are active in the first few days of life, allowing newborns to imitate the facial gestures (like smiling, opening their mouths, or sticking their tongues out) of their parents. They allow us to learn by watching others perform a task and resonating with their emotions.

The Social Engagement System

While the basic flight-fight reaction to fear is an adequate defensive strategy for nonsocial animals, caretaking, cooperation, and sustained relationships require a volume control instead of an on-off switch. We have to stay in proximity to others, and not harm or flee from those we love, even when we are upset. Thus, in addition to the attachment system, natural selection also shaped the social engagement system or the smart vagus.[9] Connecting the brain with the heart, lungs, and facial muscles (among other structures), the complex nerves that make up the vagal system allow us to modulate bodily and emotional reactions in a prosocial manner.

The *tone* of the vagus refers to the system's ability to regulate levels of arousal, including activity in our bodily organs, especially the heart. Children with poor vagal tone have difficulty regulating their emotions in stressful situations, making it difficult for them to maintain attention and sustain a shared focus of attention with others. As adults, good vagal tone allows us to become upset, anxious, or angry with loved ones without withdrawing or becoming physically aggressive.

The Social Motivation System

The social motivation system includes the neurochemicals that draw us to one another and regulate behavior such as pair bonding, social dominance, and caretaking. The most primitive neurochemicals involved in social motivation are oxytocin and vasopressin, which are associated with mating, reproduction, and caretaking. During attachment, initial bonding is driven by oxytocin and vasopressin in both mother and child. As we grow, dopamine and norepinephrine associate social interactions with feelings of happiness and excitement.

When a mother and child are separated, oxytocin levels plummet in both of them, causing distress. Interacting with his newborn results in lower levels of testosterone in the father, making him calmer and less aggressive. Over time, secure attachment schemas are shaped by the long series of positive experiences stored in attachment circuitry and a complex activations of these social neurochemicals. Later in life, positive relationships, and even the thought of the people we love, come to regulate the activation of this rewarding biochemistry.[10]

The Stress Regulation System

The hypothalamic-pituitary-adrenal (HPA) axis is the central communication system involved in the body's response to stress. It also converts the perception of danger into hormonal messengers that activate the body's fight-flight reaction. This system evolved to respond to brief stress and then quickly return to homeostasis. In conditions of chronic stress, the HPA system stays activated and can damage the body and the brain by sustaining high levels of cortisol.

Chronically high levels of cortisol inhibit the protein synthesis necessary for neuronal maintenance, brain building, learning, and proper immunological functioning. Because relationships regulate HPA activation, the calmer, safer, and more supportive our social world, the better regulated our stress-response system. This may be the key explanation for why those with more positive relationships learn better, stay healthier, and live longer.

Much research suggests that genes serve as templates to organize the general structure of the brain and trigger sensitive periods of development. As we develop, the epigenetic process called transcription translates our experience into neural material, allowing us to adapt to our particular environment. Through the biochemical alchemy of template and transcription genetics, experience becomes flesh, love takes material form, and our relationships with others become a part of our inner worlds.

THE SURVIVAL OF THE NURTURED
AND THE NURTURING

Grandchildren are God's way of compensating us for
growing old.

Mary H. Waldrip

Today, it is obvious that children need to be held, talked to, and loved. Not very long ago, even doctors thought relationships to be superfluous to our well-being. For example, in an effort to keep children from contracting and spreading disease, doctors at orphanages ordered children to be separated from one another, and direct contact with nursing and other staff was kept to an absolute minimum. While fewer children died of infectious diseases, the death rate remained so high that, for the sake of efficiency, doctors signed death certificates along with admission forms when children first arrived. This is one of the costs of thinking of humans as separate beings instead of seeing them as embedded within relationships.

In the years that followed, loss of vitality seen in orphaned and abandoned children came to be labeled as depression, hospitalism, or failure to thrive. It was observed in London orphanages during World War II and in American hospitals where parents were limited to visiting their children one hour per week during long hospital stays. A more severe form of the same phenomenon occurred more recently in Romanian orphanages. It is now obvious that children rely on interactions not only to build their brains but for their very survival.

A half century ago, a theory of aging known as *disengagement* suggested that older people naturally withdraw from their social network as they prepare to die.[11] We now understand that the need for positive attachment and meaningful interactions doesn't fade with age. A wealth of data links the amount and quality of social support to better physical and emotional health at any age. The dawning awareness of the importance of attachment in early childhood has been a century-long revelation, yet we often remain blind to its importance later in life.

Attachment is a lifelong process of engagement and reengagement as we adapt to changing roles, situations, and social resources. Those who make a greater social investment receive enhanced well-being in return. Building young brains and sustaining older ones through bonding and attachment is a naturally occurring reciprocal exchange in our social economy.

PARENTS AND GRANDPARENTS

Second thoughts are ever wiser.

Euripides

Parents and grandparents begin to forge a relationship with the next generation from the moment of conception. Early pulses of attachment are triggered by grainy ultrasound images, fantasies about what the baby will look like, and the kicks and tugs of prenatal exercise. After birth, shared sights, sounds, and smells deepen bonds as parents, grand-parents, and children become woven together into a superor-ganism called the family. These powerful visceral, sensory, and emotional connections serve as the core of lifelong attachments as our brains take in those closest to us as parts of ourselves. The tight swaddling of infancy slowly transforms into preschool and playdates, school trips and sleepovers, handing over the keys to the car, and eventually helping our offspring move into homes of their own. During this decades-long process, an ever-present dialogue between children and their family members creates narratives that help them find meaning in life.

Parents and grandparents often find themselves at odds. Some think parenting is teaching a set of rules that will help children to succeed in society, while others say it is an exer-cise in indulgence where children make the rules to which parents adapt. No matter where you fall between these two extremes, parenting is a constant challenge. We have to simultaneously socialize our children while encouraging their individuality, and provide structure and rules while being loving and playful. Children need to be allowed to express their feelings, be helped to put them into words, and create a story of their experiences.

Getting to know another person well, especially our own children, can be a real challenge. Sure, we can know some-one's likes and dislikes; we might even get good at guessing what they might be feeling. But ultimately, everything we know about someone else is influenced by our own needs and personal biases, some conscious, most not. With strangers, obvious differences and clear boundaries serve as reminders that we need to be wary of our assumptions, but with someone as close as our own children, boundaries usually blur. Young parents may have an especially difficult time discovering where they end and their children begin.

Our unconscious conflicts and needs seem to project most powerfully onto those in whom we have our largest emotional investments, especially our children and grandchildren. As living extensions of our bodies, hearts, and egos, they activate our fears and fantasies and stir up our inner demons. It can take years for parents to realize that their children are separate individuals with their own strengths and weaknesses, likes and dislikes, and hopes and dreams.

All too often, I've seen parents damage or destroy relationships with their children because they cannot fully accept that they are separate and unique individuals. So when I am asked to offer my "expert" opinion on parenting, I usually respond, "After giving them as much love as you can, you need to remember that your children are not you. Each of us is an experiment of nature that needs to discover its own expression. As parents, our job is to help our children by providing them with the emotional and material resources that allow them to discover themselves." Easier said than done.

We often bring the pain, fear, and trauma of our youth into our relationships with others, especially our children. There are situations in which our own childhoods can interfere with parenting and where the mitigating presence of grandparents and other wise, caring elders can be especially important. The fact that the construction of the human brain is shaped by social relationships has widespread implications. My hope is that as the evidence of the impact of early experience mounts, it will become clear that we need to invest more in our children and our children's children. I suspect that this growth in awareness will accompany a parallel appreciation for the need to keep people of all ages connected for the benefit of elders, children, and those in between.

3

Sustaining the Social Brain:
A New Look

*The most complicated thing in the universe is the
collective of human brains and their psychological
processes that make up human culture.*

—Henry Plotkin

As we have already seen, early nurturance
can have a profound impact on the shaping of our brains,
hearts, and minds. We have also learned that brain circuits
retain experience-dependent plasticity throughout life. In
fact, research has shown a tendency for marital partners with
insecure attachment to develop increasingly secure attachment patterns when paired with someone who is securely
attached. The same shift is also likely to occur in adoptive
children and during the course of psychotherapy.

Other studies have shown the healing value of mentors, teachers, and other adults for children who have been

neglected and abused. Even so-called hardened criminals have been known to be softened by altruistic acts and caring others. This retained plasticity in attachment circuitry makes sense given our need to attach and reattach to new people across changing circumstances throughout life.

Secure attachments first build and then maintain the health of the social brain. Further, because the networks of the social brain are central to the healthy development of the body, the social brain is also central to our physical well-being. When a grandparent interacts with a grandchild in a nurturing way, both of their brains are engaged in life-sustaining activity. While the grandparent is triggering the growth of new neurons, receptor cells, and complex neural connections in his grandchild, the grandchild, in turn, is stimulating the release of oxytocin, endorphins, and dopamine in the grandparent, having a healthy effect on his or her cognitive abilities, physical health, and longevity.

THE GRANDMOTHER GENE

> Life's most persistent and urgent question is, "What are
> you doing for others?"
>
> Martin Luther King Jr.

In the process of evolving larger, more social, and increasingly complex brains, we have grown deeply dependent on extended and sophisticated child caretaking from the adults and older children within our tribes. As part of this process, human brains became the slowest to grow and the last to show signs of aging of all the primates. This larger window of time results in greater investment in each child, increasing their chances of survival, and perpetuating our genes in into the next generation.[1]

Scientists who study our patterns of childbearing have wondered for quite a while why human females, unlike other primates, experience menopause when they still have a half to a third of their lives ahead of them.[2] One theory called the *grandmother gene hypothesis* puts forth two key reasons. The first is to avoid the risks inherent in mating and childbirth, which rise with age for both mother and child. The second is that postmenopausal women serve a greater good by being available to help nurture their grandchildren and contribute to the overall well-being of their families.[3] In essence, the grandmother gene hypothesis suggests that early menopause has been chosen by natural selection to enhance the survival rate of grandchildren and hence, the perpetuation of the grandmother's genes.

So what is the evidence for this theory? Sear, Mace, and McGregor studied subsistence tribal life in rural Gambia, where families closely depend upon one another for basic survival.[4] Their lifestyle is likely representative of the majority of our evolutionary history. The results of their research show that nutritional status, height, and the survival rate of young children were significantly correlated with the presence of postmenopausal maternal grandmothers. The presence of fathers, paternal grandmothers, or other male kin had a negligible impact on either the nutritional status or survival rates of offspring. Similar findings have been obtained in studies of different groups in Tanzania, Canada, Finland, and the United States.[5]

Historical records from Tokugawa Japan (1671–1871) revealed that grandmothers offered the greatest protection against child mortality at age two.[6] This was the general age of weaning when mothers turned their attention to the conception and birth of their next child. The researchers hypothesized that the availability of the grandmother at this time increased the child's chances of obtaining the attention and nutrition he or she needed to survive and thrive. Of course, the benefit of receiving the care and attention of any particular grandmother is related to her motivation and caretaking abilities.[7]

NURTURANCE AND LONGEVITY

What a bargain grandchildren are! I give them my loose change, and they give me a million dollars worth of pleasure.

Gene Perret

So far our focus has been on the advantages in health and survival bestowed by the presence of the maternal grandmother.

But as highly interdependent creatures with interdependent brains, it would make great sense that the health and longevity of our brains would be influenced by our active involvement in all our relationships. Is it possible that women have a longer life span than men because they are traditionally the ones who provide most of the child care? Could taking care of others be good medicine?

Some interesting evidence that may support a connection between childcare and longevity comes from looking at parenting behaviors across different species of primates. A longevity advantage for females does exist in gorillas, orangutans, and humans, species where females are the primary caretakers. On the other hand, in species such as the owl and titi monkeys, where the male is the primary caretaker of infants, males tend to survive longer. Among Goeldi monkeys who share equally in child care, the genders have equal life spans.

Given the amount of evidence supporting the beneficial effects of secure attachment, caretaking, human touch, and social support, it is plausible that caretaking, nurturing, and close contact may provide caretakers with health and survival advantages. The strength of these fundamental attachment bonds and their neurochemical and hormonal by-products may have been programmed by evolution to keep those who take care of others around longer. This may be nature showing us how interwoven we are and how important it is to take care of one another. Unfortunately, research shows that grandmothers tend to have a more positive attitude toward grandparenting than their husbands, so some men may be missing out.[8]

Early research in neuroplasticity demonstrated that rats raised in more complex and challenging environments developed larger and more sophisticated brains than those raised in bland, boring, and impoverished environments. It was also found that if the impoverished rats had offspring, caring for them stimulated brain growth to the point where their brains were like those of the rats raised in enriched environments.[9] We know these changes are not due to the hormonal by-products of pregnancy and birth because the brains of virgin rats grow when given baby rats to care for.

Human males also experience hormonal changes in response to the birth of their children that shape them to be calmer and less aggressive. These findings strongly suggest that caring for children enriches, stimulates, and challenges our brains to grow, regardless of gender and despite earlier deprivation. This may be why so many who had less than happy childhoods take great joy in being parents.

And here is something that I found surprising: Women who give birth after the age of 40 are almost four times more likely to live to be 100 years old.[10] While this is usually explained in terms of the protective nature of birth-related hormones, their enhanced longevity may be part of broader biological and psychological processes involved in intense caretaking that stimulate our brains to thrive.[11] It is a good bet that taking care of a child triggers genetic and biochemical processes in the brain and body that enhance health and slow down aging. Best of all, the elixir of attachment is all around us and free for the taking. I suspect that for every loving adult there is somewhere a lonely and neglected child in need of their attention.

A FOUNTAIN OF YOUTH?

If I had known how wonderful it would be to have grandchildren, I'd have had them first.

Lois Wyse

In their day-to-day lives, older adults often report feeling unneeded, unattractive, and unwanted. In contrast, the enthusiastic love of grandchildren and their insatiable need for interaction and attention come untainted by the prejudice of ageism. In one study, 80% of respondents reported that they enjoyed grandparenting, with 37% saying that they enjoyed it even more than parenting.[12] In a study of over 2,000 grandmothers from across the United States, 43% helped provide regular care for their grandchildren. When asked what satisfaction they received from caretaking, they reported factors such as being appreciated, the opportunity for more contact with their children, making a contribution to the family, and the opportunity to play.[13] See Table 3.1 for an impressive list of the reported positive effects of grandparenting.

Table 3.1. The Positive Effects of Grandparenting

Satisfaction and Motivation	Role Maintenance
Self-satisfaction and self-esteem [a]	A sense of doing something important [k]
Motivation: "They keep me going" [b]	Maintaining an important social role [l]
Motivation to stay fit [c]	Reason for living and a feeling of being needed [m]
Joy and pleasure [d]	The experience of being a good caretaker [n]
Decreased isolation [e]	
Decreased depression [f]	*Social Support and Connection*
Taking pleasure in the little things [g]	Social networking and social status [o]
	Social support [p]
Meaning	Emotional intimacy and fulfillment [q]
Meaning and purpose [h]	Closeness with their grandchildren [r]
A connection with the future [i]	Vitality: "They keep me young" [s]
Forming a legacy [j]	Positive emotional expression [t]

Each grandparent has an optimal range of responsibility for grandchildren that supports his or her physical and mental health. When caretaking is not elective, or occurs under duress, health benefits may begin to diminish. This is revealed in the research on those who step in to care for their grandchildren because their own children are on drugs, in prison, or suffer from AIDS. The number of grandchildren that wind up on their doorstep, as well as their emotional and physical health, play a significant role in their ability to be caretakers and benefit from these relationships.[14] These elders often have limited financial resources and may themselves suffer from physical and emotional difficulties.[15]

The remarkable thing is that even those with the greatest stress and fewest resources almost always report being enriched by caring for their grandchildren. I've had the pleasure of meeting grandparents such as these and have been inspired by their love and dedication. Below are a few quotes from published research on grandparents who are caretakers under less than optimal conditions.

Based on her own experience as a child, one grandmother stated, "I realized when I was very young how important a grandparent can be to a child, and I promised myself that I'd be a really good grandmother."[16]

The 52-year-old grandmother of a 14-year-old pregnant girl and three boys ages 1, 2, and 5 reported, "I have been diagnosed with cancer three times. I'm on chemotherapy now. Do you know that raising these kids and receiving their love is what keeps me alive? Believe it! I'm not going anywhere until they are grown and have their own families. By then I'll be raising another group of kids. It will be my third time around. I thank God for the chance."[17]

A custodial grandmother whose husband had retired said, "We (my husband and I) do things together that we never did before. . . . He never participated in raising our children. He never had time to be a parent and I asked him if he missed that and he said 'no,' and then he said . . . 'I have time this time to be involved, and I like it.' And I thought wow! . . . We are doing together what I did before."[18]

In describing her relationship with her grandchildren, a subject in another study stated, "My grandmother was the radiant angel of my childhood, and, you know, now my grandchildren are just the same. They are the part of my life that is most joyous, that gives me the most pleasure."[19]

In another study, a grandfather described his experience with his granddaughter: "To have her look up and say 'I love you.' And she'll come around once in awhile and she'll say, I'm so lucky that I have you and grandma. . . . Kelly is the coolest kid in town. . . . Everybody loves her."[20]

A Native American grandmother told an interviewer, "I am rich with years, a millionaire! I have been part of my own generation, then I watched my children's generation grow up, then my grandchildren's, and now my great-grandchildren's. Two of my great-grandchildren are becoming full-grown women now; they come visit me, and will remember me. Now, I ask you, how much more can a woman expect?"[21]

The breakdown of multigenerational families, increased mobility, and unbridled consumerism have devalued or eliminated many of our elders' traditional roles and contributions to society. The same culture that brings us increased longevity via public health and advances in medical science also isolates its elders. For many, the combination has resulted in longer lives with less purpose or meaning. At the same time, the gap between the nurturance children need and what their harried, distracted, and overworked parents are able to provide is expanding. The answer for many of the parents that I've worked with is to keep their children as harried and distracted as they are with endless activities geared toward making them more competitive as adults. Thus, the cycle continues to the next generation.

Many, including myself, feel that our values have gone off course and that we need to bring some peace and sanity back to everyday life. A part of the solution may be to re-create tribes in ways that fit modern life for connection and nurturance. Instead of putting our elders out to pasture, we might learn to harness the experience, affection, and time they have to offer. Continuing to embrace them as part of our family constellation offers a practical and moral solution to both problems.

OVERVIEW AND A NEW LOOK

For the unlearned, old age is winter; for the learned it is the season of the harvest.

                                        The Talmud

Thus far I've tried to establish the case for the brain as a social organ that survives and thrives through stimulating interpersonal interactions. As we have seen, young brains are built, shaped, and regulated by the brains of their care-takers. Plenty of evidence also attests to the fact that these same interactions are essential throughout life in order to maintain the health and well-being of our minds and bodies. This is, in essence, the social context in which we have evolved for millions of years and that our brains have been shaped to thrive in. Thus, for older adults, grandparenting, mentoring, and contributing to the lives of others may be as important as loving touch is for a young child.

The recipe for a healthy aging brain appears to be a life that maximizes social inclusion and optimizes challenge. These two ingredients appear central to the health and well-being of body, brain, and spirit. In the chapters to come, we continue exploring these concepts, using research in the neurobiology of aging, gender differences, the role of storytelling for both brain and culture, and the origins and importance of wisdom. Through this research we will explore the fabric of biological, psychological, and social factors that shape and reshape the brain. Further, since our brains change with our social roles and obligations, we will explore how the aging brain changes as a reflection of our changing social priorities at each stage of life.

From a neurological perspective, aging leads to increased participation of both cerebral hemispheres in problem solving, maturation of systems of emotional regulation, and maintenance of the neural networks involved in attachment and bonding. It also facilitates a developmental shift from neural systems dedicated to new learning to those involved in acquired knowledge and expert skills and biological changes conducive to more flexible gender role responsibilities. Psychologically, aging contributes to better decision-making, problem-solving abilities, emotional regulation, and a desire to transmit knowledge to the next generation.

Healthy aging allows for nurturing and mentoring relationships to increase in importance with a decrease in competition for men and increased assertiveness for women. Aging also leads to us to place an increased importance on being of value to others, maintaining age-appropriate leadership roles, initiating adolescents into adulthood, and sharing wisdom through mentorship and storytelling.

These brain-based changes will help us gain a new perspective on aging, one that combines a traditional understanding of the role of elders with current research and our changing society. My hope is to provide an alternative view of the maturing brain that is more useful, nurturing, and life affirming for people of all ages.

Part
Two

The Social Brain
Across the Life Span

The Life of the Brain

Beware of false knowledge; it is more dangerous than ignorance.

—George Bernard Shaw

THE MYTH ABOUT OUR BRAIN'S JOURNEY THROUGH life is a sad tale of decline; this turns out to be wrong. In addition to the complexity of the brain's structure and organization, age-related changes are also influenced by past experience, education, physical and emotional health, and the task at hand.[1] A deeper and more sophisticated look into the human brain reveals a universe of interacting neural networks and millions of connecting fibers. In fact, the brain is a sophisticated government of specialized systems that combine to perform increasingly complex tasks as we mature.

Depending on what you are doing (e.g., looking, walking, talking), different neural networks become activated and engaged, each with their own areas of expertise, gender differences, and pattern of age-related change. The brain is not a monolithic structure, and it changes during our lifetimes in complex ways; some skills and abilities improve, and some get worse, while others remain the same. Research with healthy older adults usually reveals better memory functioning than our prejudices would lead us to expect.[2] Let's begin with some basics of how the brain learns.

MEMORY AND LEARNING

> By the time you're 80 years old you've learned everything.
> You only have to remember it.
>
> George Burns

Our ability to learn and remember is dependent upon modifications of the brain's architecture and chemistry in a process known as *neural plasticity*. *Plasticity* is a general term describing the ability of the nervous system to change in response to experience.[3] Neural plasticity also includes the growth of new neurons (*neurogenesis*) and the strengthening of the connections between neurons, known as *long-term potentiation*. Learning depends upon many layers of biochemical processes that support and maintain the brain's ability to react to and store information from new experience.[4] In this manner, the architecture of our brain becomes a physical manifestation of our experiences.

Whether an infant is learning to find her thumb, a high

school student is studying history, or a grandparent is learning to use e-mail for the first time, the same neuroplastic processes occur. There is solid evidence in both animals and humans that learning triggers the brain to grow. When animals are raised in complex and challenging environments, their brains grow larger and have larger neurons, more synapses (connections among the neurons), and greater amounts of neurotransmitters and growth hormones.[5]

Research with animals has shown that new learning has the ability to mend earlier deficits. For example, adult rats exposed to training, stimulation, and enriched environments have demonstrated a reversal of earlier nervous system damage and genetically based learning deficits.[6] These sorts of positive changes have also been seen in the recovery behaviors of neglected children who are adopted into loving families. These findings speak to the marvelous flexibility of the mammalian nervous system and suggest that the challenges we take on later in life can have a profoundly positive impact on our brains.

THE LIFE OF THE FRONTAL LOBES

Long whiskers cannot take the place of brains.

Russian proverb

Theories that focus on the loss of cognitive abilities as we grow older point to the frontal lobes as the main culprit. This perspective is based in studies that show greater neural loss, decreased activation, and less dopamine availability in the frontal lobes with age.[7] But as I mentioned earlier, the brain is made up of a complex government of systems, and the frontal lobes are no exception. Let's focus on the front-most portion of the frontal lobes, known as the prefrontal cortex.

The prefrontal cortex can be divided into two general regions—those on the top and sides (dorsal and lateral), and those on the bottom and in between the two hemispheres (orbital and medial). Let's call these two regions the dorsolateral prefrontal cortex (DLPFC) and the orbitomedial prefrontal cortex (OMPFC), which you'll remember from an earlier chapter. Each area connects with many other regions of the brain to perform a wide variety of tasks.

The DLPFC connects with the rest of the cortex and the hippocampus to combine attention, sensory information, imagination, and problem solving. This is one of the primary systems in the human brain that appears to differentiate us from other primates. As I mentioned earlier, the OMPFC participates in networks with the amygdala, which organizes emotional processing, fear regulation, attachment, and the experience of self. The communication between the DLPFC and OMPFC allows us to integrate thinking with feeling and to link our inner experience with the outer world.

The DLPFC, which arose later in our evolutionary history, develops slowly over the first two decades of life and begins to decline in our late 20s. In stark contrast,

Orbital Medial Prefrontal Cortex

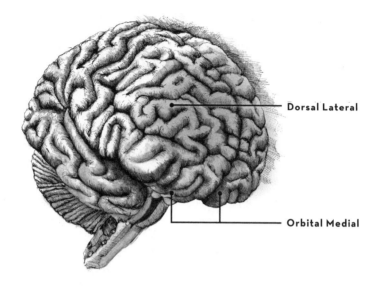

Dorsal Lateral

Orbital Medial

the OMPFC evolved much earlier, develops earlier in life, and is maintained throughout life. So while we find it harder to remember new information as we progress through adulthood, the strength of our attachment to others stays as strong as ever as our emotional stability and self-knowledge increase.

When we look more closely, we find that age-related deficits in cognitive testing are generally those dependent on the DLPFC, not the OMPFC.[8] Everyday problem solving and verbal abilities seem to improve, while performance on pencil-and-paper tests reliant on speed and new learning declines after middle age.[9] So while it's true that we don't do as well on tasks of working memory over time, our emotional and relational abilities—which cognitive psychologists almost never measure—actually get better. The same thing is true for memory. We generally think of memory as a single function, but, in fact, we have many different forms of memory that are processed in separate neural networks. For example, you may not remember a phone number, but your hand might maintain the memory for the set of movements required to press the correct numbers. Another good example is that older adults are as good at remembering faces as the young but not as good at remembering their names.[10] This is because the memory for faces involves the OMPFC, which is maintained with age, while the memory for words relies on the DLPFC.

The two general categories of memory are explicit and implicit. Explicit memory is best described as the realm of the DLPFC—conscious memory for names, places, and events. Implicit memories, the specialty of the OMPFC, do not require conscious awareness and may include early attachment experiences and trauma. Another kind of implicit memory that doesn't require conscious reflection is procedural memories such as knowing how to ride a bicycle or play a musical instrument. In contrast to explicit memory, procedural and emotional memory are relatively unimpacted by aging because they are organized in systems that don't experience age-related decline.[11] The take-home message is that whenever someone is talking about changes in memory, we have to ask, "Memory for what?"

STRESS AND MEMORY

The mind is its own place, and in itself, can make a heaven hell, a hell of heaven.

John Milton

J. B. S. Haldane, the founder of the fields of biochemistry and genetics, examined the problem of aging in his book *New Paths in Genetics*.[12] Haldane proposed that aging results from neglect on the part of natural selection. That is, aging is an accumulation of destructive genes (such as those for Huntington's disease) that escape the knife of natural selection because they impact us after our childbearing years.[13] Eleven years later George Williams suggested that aging is the cost of the energy required for earlier survival and reproduction.[14] Neither of these theories has found consistent support.

As far as anyone knows, there is no biological mandate for just how long an organism can live.[15] The longevity of any species appears to be the product of thousands of genetic, biological, and environmental variables. Thus, life spans vary from species to species; rats live for about 30 months, and humans live 70 to 80 years, while trees can live for centuries. There are even a number of single-celled organisms that are thought to be immortal. In fact, most of the neurons we have when we die were present when we were born and are still functioning just fine. Neurons most often die as a result of inadequate oxygen and nutrition or the buildup of internal waste products that interfere with their functioning. Neurons do not appear to have a definite life span.

Scientists have found that the longevity of certain species can be quickly modified. Removing the adrenal gland (and the stress hormones it generates) of the king salmon doubles its life span from 4 to 8 years, while the introduction of a specific parasite on its gills can increase its life span to 13 years.[16] In both cases, the biochemistry of the salmon is changed in ways that decrease the negative impact of stress hormones on its physical well-being.

The impact of stress on humans is well documented. A dramatic example is the decline in life expectancy in Russia since the fall of communism in 1990 and the ensuing years of chaos and uncertainty.[17] Thus, it is not just our genes that determine our life span, but factors such as culture, lifestyle, the quality of our relationships, and anything else that causes or decreases stress. The question of human longevity reaches beyond our genes to our language, our culture, and the minds with whom we are linked.

Our more recently evolved cortex sits atop and is interwoven with the primitive neural systems for danger (fight-flight) conserved from our reptilian ancestors. A key component of this system is the release of cortisol, a hormone involved in shifting our functioning from long-term maintenance to a focus on immediate survival. While cortisol makes energy available for emergency situations, it also results in a shutdown of the protein synthesis required for both neuroplasticity and immunological functioning. It is especially toxic to the brain's center for new learning, the hippocampus.[18]

Cortisol triggers hippocampal neurons to work harder and harder until they actually run out of energy, collapse, and die.[19] In addition, since cortisol impedes the synthesis of protein in the brain and body, stress may result in decreased neurogenesis and neural growth.[20] In either case, the result might be deficits in our ability to fight off disease and learn new information.[21] This process is especially detrimental to children and adolescents as it impedes their neurological, psychological, and social development.

The hippocampus is not only vulnerable to cortisol, but also to lack of oxygen. Mountain climbers and divers who experience periods of lower oxygen availability demonstrate hippocampal shrinkage and memory deficits. A natural part of aging is a decrease in the integrity and efficiency of the small capillaries that bring oxygen to the brain, which would contribute to hippocampal cell loss. Thus, some memory loss can be caused by vascular deterioration.[22]

Although a decline in explicit memory is a common feature of aging, we have no way of knowing whether it is necessary. The hippocampus does not appear to automatically lose neurons based specifically on aging. In fact, the size of temporal lobe memory areas is maintained until very late in life.[23] It appears that deficits in learning and memory are the result of multiple processes that can damage hippocampal structure or impede its proper functioning.[24]

COGNITIVE RESERVE

Old age is like everything else. To make a success of it,
you've got to start young.

Theodore Roosevelt

Performance on any specific cognitive task requires the activation of specialized areas and the inhibition of others that might hinder efficient processing. From adolescence onward, we tend to use more and more of our brains to solve problems. It has been shown that older subjects activate regions of social and emotional processing even when they are asked to engage in tasks that don't require them. This leads them to perform more slowly and less well than their younger counterparts.[25] This evolutionary age-related bias may lead older folks to use more of their brains than necessary for more straightforward tasks.[26]

Declines in basic sensory, motor, and balance functions also take a toll on brain functioning. The more attention it takes to navigate the environment—seeing through clouded lenses and walking on creaky limbs—the less we have available for cognitive functioning in other areas.[27] This may be why older adults perform as well as younger adults on some memory tasks but require more time, as previously automatic processes come to require greater effort.[28] In fact, as we age, tests of visual memory result in an increased activation of brain areas not activated in younger adults.[29] Because the neural networks involved in cognitive processing are interwoven with those dedicated to sensory and motor function, age-related declines in these basic abilities have an adverse effect on cognitive processing.

Cognitive reserve is a hypothesis that may help us understand why some older adults are better able to cope with the effects of aging and brain disease than others. The basic theory states that the more neural structure a brain has, the more complex its organization and the more resilient it will be to the negative effects of aging and injury. It is believed that the cognitive declines associated with even healthy aging are related to the gradual degeneration of dendrites, neurons, and the biochemical mechanisms that support neural health and plasticity.[30] This implies that, the more neural material you have built throughout life, the more you can afford to lose while still functioning competently.[31]

People with larger cognitive reserves are thought to be those who have had a better diet, higher-quality education, and more challenging jobs.[32] Factors such as larger brain size, early learning, and greater occupational attainment also seem to mitigate against the effects of Alzheimer's disease, traumatic injury, and the general impact of brain aging.[33] Studies have found that expected age-related intellectual decline can be halted or reversed in many older adults by increasing environmental and social stimulation.[34] The most efficient explanation would be that these experiences correlate with biological processes that enhance plasticity, creating more elaborate, complex, and flexible brains.

A number of studies, including Dr. Snowdon's research

with the sisters of Notre Dame, suggest that those who have had more education and more challenging occupations tend to have brains that age better and resist the onset and progression of dementia. Snowdon and his colleagues found that measures of cognitive function in the nuns at age 22 were associated with reduced brain weight, cerebral atrophy, and symptoms of Alzheimer's disease more than half a century later.[35] In other words, the better the nuns functioned in early adulthood, the healthier their brains were near the end of life.

About 25% of older individuals exhibiting no symptoms of Alzheimer's disease while alive show significant Alzheimer's-related brain pathology upon autopsy.[36] Individuals with more education had a significantly greater amount of plaques and tangles in their neurons yet functioned as well as others with less advanced disease.[37] This suggests that individuals with more education can sustain a greater amount of neural damage and still maintain the same level of cognitive functioning as those with less education.

Skills most dependent upon frontal functions, such as the verbal fluency and abstract thinking demanded by high-complexity occupations, appear to strongly contribute to cognitive reserve.[38] Unfortunately for me, being a college professor does not protect against brain aging, although it may slow down some of its manifestations.[39] Although cognitive reserve is thought to account for only 5% of our ability to predict brain health, building our brains through stimulating activities is something we know that we can do to support brain health.[40]

THE PRIVILEGE OF AGE

Anyone who stops learning is old, whether at 20 or 80.

Henry Ford

Age has its privileges, or so the saying goes. After raising a family, taking care of our parents, and decades of toil, we have earned the right to sit back and relax. We can say no to things that are challenging, make us uncomfortable, or require too much effort. "Let's vacation at the same place each year; it's comfortable and predictable, and we know where to find what we need. Let the kids figure out how to work the computer, surf the internet, or program a new cell phone. To hell with meeting new people—I already have enough friends."

Indeed we have earned this right, but keep in mind how the brain interprets these attitudes and behaviors: "Relax— you don't need to grow new neurons, build new dendrites, or create new connections. In fact, we can probably cut back on energy going to the brain and channel it elsewhere." There is a type of sea barnacle that is born with a brain that has only four functions: (1) direct motion in the water, (2) detect a source of food, (3) attach to a stationary object like a rock or pier, and (4) have yourself digested. That's right, the brain is a metabolically expensive organ, and if it's no longer needed, it can atrophy or, in the case of the sea barnacle, trigger a self-destruct program.

Centrally related to the privilege of age is the avoidance

of anxiety and risk taking. And while high levels of anxiety are to be avoided, moderate anxiety connected with the excitement of learning something new, meeting new people, or landing in an unfamiliar country can be especially good for your brain. In fact, mild anxiety in response to stimulating challenges serves as a signal to the brain: "Kick up neuron production, stimulate metabolism, and let's make some new connections." This positive excitement can be confused with anxiety, but it is something our brains need to stay alive. Unfortunately, many lose the ability to differentiate between positive and negative anxiety and become increasingly avoidant of any kind of challenge.

Perhaps positive arousal should be renamed "stimulation" because this is precisely the result within our brains. The brain was designed to change, so the old adage "use it or lose it" has a great deal of neural validity.[41] The aging brain retains the capacity to grow in an experience-dependent manner and has to be stimulated by environmental, relational, and internal challenges.[42] Being in a position where we have to solve problems stimulates our brains, telling them to stay alert, pay attention, learn, and grow.

Given the importance of continued bonding and attachment, one of the most important directions in which to orient our exploration is toward those around us. It is vitally important that we remain curious about who our children and grandchildren are and that we continue to play and remain open to imagination. What we have learned about neural plasticity tells us that the brain is primed to grow in states of safety, positive excitement, shared openness, and exploration. These states of mind create the flexibility that allows us to adapt to our children and help them discover their inner worlds. Attunement, secure attachment, curiosity, affect regulation, and brain plasticity walk hand in hand. This is as true in the first days of life as it is after a century. In Buddhism, what is known as *beginner's mind* is a way to look at the world as if for the first time, with interest, enthusiasm, and engagement. This may be the optimal state of mind for a healthy brain.

5

Growth and Adaptation

Aging is the neglected stepchild of the human life cycle.

—Robert Butler

THE FIRST TIME I CRADLED A HUMAN BRAIN IN MY hands, my reaction was pure fascination. I explored the convolutions of the cortex, peered deeply into the fissure separating the hemispheres, and marveled at the cerebellum nestled below. The few pounds of neurons, glial cells, and supporting tissue I was holding once contained a person's life: the sights, sounds, and smells of a culture, a memory of first love, and the last thoughts before death. The fact that a brain is capable of such things is almost beyond comprehension.

Until recently, it was assumed that brain growth ceased after childhood and that aging was synonymous with decay. The brain was also thought of as a static organ, like the heart and lungs, performing the same job in the same way from birth until death. Our brains, however, have been shaped by evolution to adapt and readapt to the ever-changing demands of our physical and social environments. Not only does the structure of the brain change throughout life, but so does the way it processes information. As we will see, many adaptations are tied to the changing social demands that we face during each phase of life.

Lifelong plasticity, the accumulation of knowledge, and the motivation to transmit wisdom to the next generations all contribute to the birth and growth of culture. While most social mammals have a three-stage life span (infant, juvenile, and adult), humans have at least five: infant, child, juvenile, adolescent, and adult.[1] In addition, current research supports the need for multiple stages of adulthood in light of our increasing longevity and an expanded focus on the complexity of modern life.

While our general focus is on older adults, the brain is best understood in the context of its development across the entire life span. In addition to looking at the changing structures and functions of the brain, we will also consider the social and emotional challenges we face in our roles as children and parents, learners and teachers, clients and therapists. Weaving together these multiple perspectives will reflect the rich tapestry of the aging process as an evolving matrix of energy, information, and relationships. Let's start at the beginning.

THE NEWBORN BRAIN

The principle activities of brains are making changes in themselves.

Marvin Minsky

Isn't it amazing that some newborn animals can stand and walk on wobbly legs within minutes of birth? Unlike us, these animals don't have the luxury of a gradual introduction to the world. They have to be ready to contribute to their own survival almost immediately by seeking shelter, finding food, or keeping up with the herd. Fortunately, our survival doesn't depend on our ability to walk, jump, run, or climb a tree on our first day. For humans, our survival depends upon our ability to attach to and be protected by those around us. If a human child is lucky enough to be born to available, sane, and healthy parents, he or she can expect many years of healthy development.

Animals that are born ready to rock and roll (or at least walk and run) rely largely on preprogrammed brains driven by deep evolutionary instincts. In stark contrast, we humans are extremely premature, highly dependent newborns whose brains are largely shaped after birth. The evolution of our social brain is revealed in reflexes to orient toward our mother, stare into her eyes, and smile to make her interested in us. We take turns making sounds, play peekaboo, and learn the cadence and melodies of communication. Freedom from fighting for physical survival allows for a long and gradual runway for development that makes ours the most highly complex brains we know of.

During early brain development, a number of simultaneous processes occur. The first is that adjacent neurons begin to connect. In this process, neurons fire together, wire together, and form functional networks, which come to organize our behaviors, thoughts, and emotions. Nature's strategy is to overproduce neurons and allow those that are unsuccessful in connecting with others to die off in a process called *apoptosis*. This neural Darwinism appears to optimize effective brain development and functioning. Apoptosis demonstrates that the normal loss of neurons is not an indication of brain disease and loss of function.

Another aspect of brain development is the emergence of connective fibers, or white matter, that link distant regions of the brain to establish complex adaptive networks. As these networks grow and interconnect with one another, electrical brain wave patterns gradually synchronize, yet another indication of brain development. The sophistication of these connections and the participation of diverse brain regions in abstract thinking and problem solving continues throughout life.

Early brain development is characterized by *sensitive periods* that are genetically programmed times of exuberant neural growth in specific brain networks in response to specific stimuli. In the first days of life, the visual cortex is stimulated by a flood of lights, edges, and colors as it begins to adapt to the newborn's physical world. During the first few months, relationships shape networks of attachment and emotional regulation. Year two ushers in an explosion of language development as the left hemisphere enters a sensitive period. It is important for healthy development that we have adequate and appropriate stimulation while we are going through sensitive periods. Although the concept of sensitive periods of neural development was initially considered to apply only during early childhood, we now know that they also occur in adolescence and most likely throughout life.

THE ADOLESCENT BRAIN

Poetry is adolescence fermented, and thus preserved.

Ortega y Gasset

Until recently, the scientific dogma was that the brain was relatively fixed after the first few years of life. It was clear that it grew larger and that we learned more information, but these changes were seen as a matter of quantity rather than quality. But when researchers began to take a closer look at adolescent brains, they were amazed by the amount of neural upheaval they found. They found considerable plasticity and reorganization taking place in the frontal lobes from the onset of puberty into the early 20s. Once this was discovered, it became obvious that the psychological and social upheavals of adolescence coincided with a previously unrecognized sensitive period of neurological maturation. This now seems obvious and has become the new dogma.

For most of our evolutionary history, humans were considered adults by their mid-teens and were expected to mate and begin to have children of their own. Consider the challenges that adolescents face. They need to establish a social identity, connect with a peer group, and create new boundaries with their families—powerful drives from our Paleolithic mandates. These challenges require reshaping of attachment bonds as they move from being passive recipients of care to caretakers. Adolescents have to break with the values and structures of their family of origin and become desirable to comrades, mates, and peers, simultaneously transferring sources of emotional security outside the immediate family.

These new demands require extensive plasticity in the prefrontal cortex to accommodate so much social upheaval and problem solving. So while your teenagers may be making you crazy, it's no picnic for them either. These radical changes in the brain parallel the sheer rawness of youth— the sudden mood swings, intense passion, and that all-encompassing feeling that you are alone in a vast and hostile world. To make things even more challenging, modern culture has prolonged childhood for an extra decade so that the impulse to be an adult slams into the expectations of conformity and obedience expected of children at home and at school.

The biological and social revolutions of adolescence are not without their dangers. Driven by rising hormones and compromised emotional regulation, the prefrontal cortex is destabilized, making judgment and insight less than stellar. What adolescents lack in perspective, they attempt to compensate for with energy, emotion, and a can-do spirit. While necessary for many of the challenges adolescents once faced as hunter-gatherers, these qualities are poorly matched to the demands of the modern world.

Adolescents become intoxicated with a feeling of invincibility while simultaneously suffering from impairments of judgment and impulse control—a toxic combination. Just check the car insurance rates for teenage drivers and how their risk of having an accident soars when they are "under the influence" of driving with their peers. The gradual decrease of insurance rates into adulthood parallels the increase in brain development that leads them to better judgment and impulse control. Those of us who marvel at how we survived adolescence cringe at the thought of our own adolescents let loose in the world.

Reward systems, such as those mediated by dopamine, also destabilize during adolescence to drive new attachments, passions, and goals. The strong drive to find their purpose and meaning makes adolescents more vulnerable to both good and bad social influences, peer pressure, and destructive cults.[2] Many become vulnerable to increased risky behaviors, eating disorders, and addictions.[3] Tobacco and alcohol companies are well aware of this vulnerability and spend vast amounts of money to convert teenagers into lifelong customers. While the sensitive period of adolescence was selected to get young people passionate about starting their own lives and contributing to the tribe, it puts them at risk in our modern world.

From adolescence through early adulthood, brain development continues with structural changes that parallel advances in language, judgment, impulse control, and emotional regulation.[4] Just as in early childhood, individual neurons continue to be eliminated as the brain's neural networks become more efficient in their functioning.[5] The brain is on its way to peak performance in areas of speed, motor coordination, and sensory acuity. Historically, these strengths contributed to tribal survival through hunting, fighting, and mating. As we near the end of adolescence and move into adulthood, enhanced communication, integration, and inhibition among different neural networks lead to increased speed of abstract functioning, and improved emotional regulation and problem-solving abilities.

THE ADULT BRAIN

Forty is the old age of youth; fifty the youth of old age.

Victor Hugo

Through our 20s, the hormonal, neural, and social upheavals of adolescence gradually settle down. The prefrontal cortex continues to mature and connect with other regions of the brain.[6] We see a more streamlined and efficient brain that performs better because of increased organization and greater hormonal and emotional stability. The dorsal and lateral regions of the prefrontal cortex and the parietal lobes mature and interconnect with the rest of the cortex, supporting higher levels of imagination and abstract thinking. We also see improvements in planning, spatial memory, and long-term memory.[7]

During young adulthood, especially in males, lateral specialization in the frontal lobes reaches its peak. This increasing specialization involves the active inhibition of brain regions in the other hemisphere that could do the same job but less efficiently.[8] This processing strategy reflects the choice by natural selection of speed over deliberation at this stage of life. Keep in mind that lateral specialization reverses later in adulthood as the brain adapts to new roles in which deep thinking is crucial and speed is not. At the beginning of adulthood, speed and efficiency trump reflection and long deliberation.

In midlife, the number of neurons within the cortex continues to decrease while subcortical structures appear to stabilize. Although neuronal loss is almost always interpreted as reflecting declining function after young adulthood, there is no definitive evidence that this is true for healthy adults. From childhood through adolescence and into young adulthood, apoptosis continues to be a normal aspect of brain maturation associated with increasing abilities.[9] The space once occupied by excess neurons becomes filled with glial cells and chemical compounds that enhance neural processing capabilities.[10] In contrast to earlier adulthood, we see increases in the volume of white matter into midlife, with a gradual decrease thereafter. This loss of white matter may have little impact or may serve to lessen the efficiency of coordination among brain regions.[11]

If this increasing participation of multiple brain regions is an adaptive strategy from childhood onward, shifts in white matter may be a functional aspect of the aging brain. Slower, more inclusive, and more thoughtful processing develops as we grow older, likely serving the increased synthetic knowledge and problem-solving abilities traditionally expected of tribal elders. In fact, when brain activity is measured by the complexity of electrical activity, there is an increase from childhood into the 60s, the highest age measured.[12] Table 5.1 summarizes the structural brain changes during midlife.

Table 5.1. Structural Changes in the Brain During Midlife

Gray Matter Changes	Effects
Decreases in the density and volume of cortical gray matter	Neural systems become more focused, specific, and efficient later in life[a]
Posterior temporal lobe volume increases until age 30, then decreases	This may reflect the initial increase and subsequent slow decline in processing and remembering external events[b]
Subcortical volume loss is much less pronounced during aging	
White Matter Changes	
Increases in volume until midlife and decreases thereafter	Subcortical structures are more stable with less emotional variation[c]
	Continuing integration of neural systems until 40-50 years of age with increases in problem solving[d]

As we shift our focus from measures of overall brain volume to specific areas and networks, we find that aging is not uniform. Generally, brain networks that evolved most recently and develop most slowly during childhood and adolescence show earlier signs of aging.[13] Remember that the dorsal and lateral areas of the prefrontal lobes (DLPFC), which continue to mature through adolescence and into our 20s, show the earliest signs of decline. White matter tracts connecting these regions to temporal and hippocampal structures show early signs of volume loss, likely contributing to decreases in short-term memory.[14] This is why for most of us, no matter how wise we may grow over the years, it gets harder to recall peoples' names, find where we parked the car, and remember that our glasses are on our heads.

Declines in executive function, explicit memory, and attention processed by the DLPFC are in stark contrast to the OMPFC systems that specialize in attachment and emotional regulation. The retention and even improvement of social judgment and empathy reflect the continued health and development of brain networks associated with the OMPFC.[15] Solid social judgment relies on the accumulation of experience, thoughtful consideration, and emotional maturity. Although there may be a decreased need for new learning and quick reactions as we age, natural selection found sustained attachment and emotional stability to be worthy of the investment the body continues to make in the social brain throughout life.

THE OLDEST OLD

*Growing old is no more than a bad habit which a busy
person has no time to form.*

André Maurois

In 1962, there were 1,500 centenarians in the United States.
By 1995, the U.S. Census Bureau counted 50,000 and predicted this number to rise to 1,000,000 by 2050.[16] By that
time, people over 85 will be the fastest-growing age group
in society. The belief that increases in the population of the
oldest old will be a drain on society is based on the idea
that they will suffer from more diseases and disabilities as
they age.

In reality, the oldest old are in pretty good shape. Many
healthy older adults show no signs of significant brain volume loss past 100 years of age.[17] The most common explanation for this phenomenon is that those people who live to
their mid-90s are particularly resistant to diseases that killed
the others in their age group. Because of their robustness,
they not only outlive others, but do so with relatively few
disabilities. Many of the oldest old, like Madame Calment,
lead active, healthy lives with short periods of illness and
infirmity before passing away.

In contrast to younger-old adults, where women are generally healthier, the oldest old are typically men who are mentally and physically healthier than women. This is a by-product

of the fact that men with dementia and other disabling illnesses tend to die from them earlier, while women survive
despite these illnesses. The first signs of this gender crossover can be seen at the age of about 80 years. In a study
at the National Institute of Aging, it was found that 44%
of the men in that age group were robust and independent
compared with only 28% of women.[18] While the currently
available data are inadequate to draw conclusions, we can
guess that the brains of the oldest old have a great deal to
teach us about positive aging.

THE EVOLUTION OF SOCIAL ANIMALS

Realize that you will live several lifetimes. You may be
one person at 20, another at 60, and another at 80.

Lena Horne

The coevolution of the human brain with caretaking, attachment, family, and culture suggests that our social roles and
responsibilities should be a central focus in understanding
healthy aging. Our increasing understanding of how epigenetics translates experience into neural structure suggests
that our experiences trigger many brain-building processes
throughout the life span. For example, as many as 540 genes
related to brain-based events have been shown to have different activation patterns at different times of life.[19] It is logical
to assume that the expression of some of these genes may be
triggered by the brain's response to changes in social roles

and relationships. In other words, our biologies may utilize the flexibility of transcription genetics to maximize functioning in response to changing social challenges throughout life.

Just as presenting a virgin rat with a rat pup stimulates areas of her brain to grow, being needed, respected, and admired activates neural plasticity and brain growth in older human adults. Research with zebra finches has shown that their ability to learn their songs is enhanced when exposed to live singing birds versus tape recordings of the same birdsong.[20] Some are actually unable to learn from tape recordings and require positive interactions with a teacher to stimulate the brain.[21] Similarly, there is something about positive relationships that help humans to learn. The opposite is also true—have you ever tried to learn something new in the presence of a critical onlooker?

A caring, supportive other creates a state of mind and body that primes our internal biology for new learning—call it a pro-plasticity state of mind. We often see that high-risk children and adolescents who eventually have successful lives had at least one person who took an interest in them—a mentor, teacher, or coach—someone who gave them time, believed in them, and encouraged their success. This is not to be taken lightly; it points to the fact that, like birds learning their song, we may learn better face to face and heart to heart. If social interactions and neuroplasticity are synergistic, it is clear why elders who become isolated are more likely to lose cognitive functions. On the other hand, those that remain connected, challenged, and needed are far more likely to remain vital and alive. Isolation and lack of stimulation are the enemies of a healthy brain at any age.

In addition to adaptations to changing social demands, it is also likely that we need to adjust to the changing realities of our bodies. Let's assume that as we age, the body is less able to produce energy. Less energy presents an adaptational challenge—how shall resources be allocated to optimize functioning? Like someone operating an energy grid, decisions have to be made concerning where to channel energy, where to cut it off, and where to turn it down. Hospitals and airports may have high priorities, while casinos and playgrounds end up in the dark. Could a similar adaptational challenge face the brain during aging?

Let's say that our brains have to make do with 10% less energy each decade after we turn 40. Where would the cuts be made and how would the remaining energy be deployed? Obviously we would have to maintain those vital brain stem functions that keep us alive. These circuits would be like our hospitals and airports. Other than these life-sustaining processes, all other circuits would be subject to energy cuts. With age, competent brains may adjust to changes in energy availability by diminishing the functioning of some less vital networks and employing alternate ways of processing information.

By midlife we have usually mated, built a nest, and created a foundation for our sustained survival. Given that we have traditionally lived in close social groups where younger people were present to do the hunting, gathering, and fighting, perhaps older adults were shaped for different roles and contributions to the tribe. Maintaining resources dedicated to attachment, affect regulation, and caretaking supports continued social interaction, nurturance, and participation in the social economy. As we will see, the bias toward retaining old memories and the impulse to tell stories points to the role of the elder as the storehouse of culture, memory, and wisdom.

Think about the elder's need to connect and contribute and the child's need to be seen, loved, and encouraged. This is a naturally occurring cycle of birth and renewal that is often missed in modern society. The loss of the extended family has taken with it millions of years of natural selection that contributes to the development and well-being of all generations. The atomization of families may contribute to many problems, from more physical illnesses to school failure, for which we turn to drugs, consumerism, and other distractions in order to cope.

6

Two Brains: Many Possibilities

The family is one of nature's masterpieces.
—George Santayana

As you already know, our brains are divided into right and left hemispheres. For many animals, the two halves of the brain are essentially identical, providing redundant systems as backup in case of injury. Dolphins and many birds, for example, sleep one hemisphere at a time, allowing them to remain in constant motion and vigilant to threat.[1] Primates, on the other hand, have followed an alternative evolutionary path where the hemispheres differentiate in both their structure and function. And if that isn't complicated enough, men's and women's brains and hemispheres are different and follow somewhat separate developmental paths. Both lateral specialization and gender differences are important aspects of the evolution of our social brains.

The movement away from identical hemispheres was likely driven by the need for more neural territory once heads had grown as large as possible given the size limitations of the birth canal. More neural space allows for the development of new skills and abilities, increasing speed of processing and behavioral and cognitive flexibility.[2] One aspect of increased hemispheric specialization has been an increase in the size of the corpus callosum, the primary communication pathway between the left and right hemispheres.[3]

NATURE'S ASYMMETRY

By denying scientific principles, one may maintain any paradox.

Galileo Galilei

Over a century ago, the Catholic Church chided Paul Broca for suggesting that language was lateralized to the left hemisphere, assuring him that God would not have made us asymmetrical. Nature, it appears, had other plans. In fact, the most obvious difference between the hemispheres in most of us (primarily right handers) is the dominance of the left for spoken language and the right for bodily and emotional processing. For the first 18 months of life, the right hemisphere experiences a growth spurt as we develop attachments and begin to build structures responsible for emotional regulation. Meanwhile, the development of the left hemisphere is held back, reserving space for language abilities to emerge during the second year of life.

In line with their functional specializations, the right and left hemispheres process information somewhat differently. The left is more linear and sequential (good for language and logic) while the right can simultaneously analyze multiple elements of the same phenomenon (good for visual and imaginative processes). This is why neurons in the right are more intricately connected, and neurons in the left are organized into linear pathways.[4] Although the hemispheres have different specialties, they cooperate for most tasks, each contributing its own set of abilities.

Interestingly, we are finding that throughout development, the nature and extent of the relationship between the hemispheres appears to change. During the first few years of life, the hemispheres operate in a relatively independent manner. As the connecting fibers between them mature, coordination and integration increase. As we move into adolescence and young adulthood, there is considerable hemispheric specialization in many memory and spatial functions.[5]

Beyond young adulthood, there appears to be a reduction of hemispheric asymmetry in the prefrontal lobes for tasks of memory and sensory processing. These shifts result in a processing strategy that can be just as accu-

Cycles of Organization in the Cebral Hemispheres

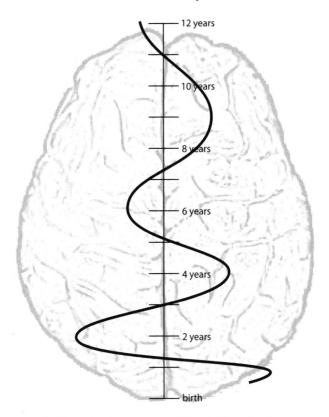

12 years

10 years

8 years

6 years

4 years

2 years

birth

Left Hemisphere   **Right Hemisphere**

rate, but slower and more effortful. As the brain continues to mature, changing activation patterns across regions of each hemisphere reflect complex adjustments in how we process information.[6]

ONGOING ADAPTATION

*Little knowledge is not to be compared with great
knowledge, nor a short life with a long life.*

                               Chuang Tsu

Despite neuroscience's historic pessimism about the aging
brain, the rest of us have noticed that age corresponds with
an increasing fund of knowledge, a deeper comprehension
of meaning, and a preservation or even improvement of narrative abilities.[7] Healthy older adults actually demonstrate
a greater complexity of brain wave patterns reflecting the
increased distribution and coordination of cortical activation.[8] Interestingly, high-performing older adults show bilateral activation, while lower-performing older adults use the
same lateralized strategies as younger adults.[9] These findings
suggest that as we age, a greater number of better-organized
networks are participating in abstract reasoning and problem solving.

For most of human history, the lives of children, parents, and grandchildren were unchanging. Older adults had
little new to learn but much to teach. And prior to the
relatively new invention of written language, older individuals were the vessels of knowledge, history, and culture.
Assuming a stable environment, frontal systems involved
in new learning were less vital, and a holistic understanding of situations was far more important than speed. Thus,

the way the brain ages appears to have been shaped by the needs of the group within an oral culture.[10] Holding multiple perspectives in mind requires widespread neural participation that accesses thinking, feeling, past learning, and present realities.

This brings up an important question—could what is usually interpreted as compensation for declining function provide older adults with the kind of neural network integration that contributes to the attainment of wisdom? As we will see in later chapters, definitions of wisdom all seem to include a blending of intellect, emotional sensitivity, empathy, and practical knowledge. Bilateral participation supports the advanced social abilities traditionally sought out in tribal elders. This stands in contrast to those we think of as "intelligent" but lack the ability to connect with and understand the feelings and needs of others.

Increased neural participation may take more time but also provides us with more and better-quality information on which to base our decisions. It is not surprising that taking more time before responding to questions is usually experienced by others as the gift of reflection and thought. Wisdom emerges from deep thought, the inclusion of multiple perspectives, and concern for those with whom it is shared. While there is no argument that age-related declines in memory and processing speed do exist, older adults may be well served by taking more time to consider the multiple aspects of a problem.

OF MEN AND WOMEN

Women who seek to be equal to men lack ambition.

Albert Einstein

Just as natural selection has shaped the right and left hemi-spheres to play specialized and complementary roles in neural processing, males and females have also been shaped for complementary contributions to the social economy. Their bodies, brains, and biochemistries have been tuned to meet the demands of gender-specific roles.[11] Sociologists often describe men as instrumental and women as expressive. Instrumental men focus on the outside world, solve problems, and attain goals related to hunting, fighting, or competing in the rat race. Expressive women stay closer to home, tending to hearth and hearts.[12]

In some cultures, these roles are shifting and gender roles and identification are coming to be seen as existing on a spectrum, but for most of the world and through much of our evolutionary histories, these general tendencies have bred true. Keep in mind that our brains are essentially Paleolithic, meaning they haven't changed much in tens of thousands of years, while culture can transform in a few generations.

Differences between males and females in cognitive and emotional processing emerge early in life and persist into adulthood. Genetic inheritance, hormonal differences, and cultural biases result in male and female brains that are quite different. From the moment of conception, our bodies and brains begin to differentiate based on the presence of an X or Y chromosome. These differences set off a cascade of reactions that guide our behaviors, determine our life histories, and shape our brains. It has been said that females are the norm and males are the genetic experiment, implying that males are a modification of the basic female model. Males do seem to be more fragile, suffering higher rates of spontaneous abortion, retardation, and learning disabilities as well as more age-related indications of neural degeneration.[13]

When it comes to spoken language, the brains of men and women are organized a bit differently. Women have a greater density of neurons in the planum temporale, a region of the temporal lobes specializing in language.[14] When given a spatial memory task, women use more verbal strategies and show greater activation in their left hippocampus, which supports language functions. Men, on the other hand, process visual-spatial information more directly without the mediation of language.[15] Gender differences in the way we process information parallel differences in gray matter density, blood flow, metabolism, and patterns of neural activation.[16]

There are also gender differences in the fibers connecting the hemispheres. The corpus callosum and two smaller structures linking left and right hemispheres are significantly larger in women.[17] In males, the corpus callosum increases in size until age 20 and then begins to decline, while in females it continues to grow until midlife.[18] Females also have a higher ratio of gray matter in the corpus callosum, suggestive of more integrated processing.[19] All of these differences between the brains of men and women point to what we all know—men and women experience the world and express themselves in different ways.

What specific skills and processing abilities support success in traditional gender roles? Men are better at hand-eye coordination and hitting targets with thrown objects, while women are superior in abilities related to foraging, verbal communication, and emotional attunement. Men tend to excel at tasks of mathematical reasoning and navigation over large distances, while women are better at tasks requiring semantic memory, language, mathematical calculations, and precise manual dexterity. All of these differences are likely embedded within gender role differentiation from our long history as hunter-gatherers.[20]

The fight-flight reaction, an essentially male survival strategy, mobilizes the brain and body to exert physical energy for combat or evasion. Increases in respiration and energy availability and enhanced sensory processing occur in the service of actively confronting danger. Given that women are generally smaller and slower than men and tend to have their young in tow, a fight-flight strategy is often not wise. Women have traditionally survived less through strength than by forming affiliations in a "tend and befriend" strategy.[21] For humans and other mammals, females with more social skills and larger social networks have a higher likelihood of survival for themselves and their children.[22]

SEX HORMONES

*It's a funny thing that when a man hasn't anything on earth
to worry about, he goes off and gets married.*

Robert Frost

Estrogen and testosterone are sex hormones that shape
brain growth and contribute to determining the cognitive
strengths of each gender for specific reproductive and social
roles.[23] Although much of our understanding of estrogen
and testosterone is based on animal studies, the increasing
medical use of hormone supplementation is expanding our
knowledge of how they function in humans, especially their
impact on the brain. Let's begin with estrogen.

Estrogen receptors have been discovered in diverse
regions of the brain, where it both enhances learning and
serves a protective purpose in injury and aging.[24] It protects
neurons from cell death and supports myelin formation and
maintenance.[25] Estrogen increases neurochemical activity in
the synapses and results in greater branching of neurons
supportive of new learning and works against oxidative processes that damage neurons over time. Given the strong link
between estrogen, brain health, and neural longevity, estrogen is obviously more than a sex hormone.[26]

The connection between estrogen and the hippocampus is an ancient one, and the hippocampus still responds
robustly to estrogen.[27] Surges of estrogen triggered by childbearing turbocharge the hippocampus to support the spatial

learning and memory required for finding, storing, and retrieving food. In fact, as estrogen levels rise and fall during the phases of the menstrual cycle, so do women's motor and perceptual skills.[28] A single administration of testosterone has been shown to enhance visuospatial abilities in young women, while testosterone replacement therapy in men of any age improves muscle strength, sexual functioning, mood, and brain functioning.[29] In a 10-year study of over 400 men, higher levels of testosterone were positively correlated with better memory, visual-motor functioning, and an overall reduced rate of decline and the development of Alzheimer's disease.[30]

"NOW SHE WANTS ME TO DO THE DISHES"

Men are taught to apologize for their weaknesses, women for their strengths.

Lois Wyse

During early and middle adulthood, gender roles related to reproduction, child care, and basic survival are front and center. But as men age, the demand for them to be protectors, hunters, and warriors gradually declines. In healthy aging, flexibility in social roles increases—men may assume the role of diplomat, peacekeeper, or nurturer, while women become more likely to engage in activities outside of the home and take on leadership roles. In other words, later in life, each gender can take on more of the aspects usually associated with the opposite sex.

The emotional adjustments necessary for retirement often catch men by surprise. Some adhere so rigidly to the role of the stoic breadwinner that they find themselves completely lost when it comes to relaxation or trying something new. Making it more difficult is the fact that men are often socialized to believe that roles within the family and community are demeaning, less serious, and less important than their past careers. Relentlessly driving themselves for decades, they have never given a thought to what their first morning of retirement will be like. And while some replace careers with hobbies without skipping a beat and others discover they enjoy relaxing, still others spin out of control. These changes present new challenges and new opportunities.

For this last group of men, retirement is a series of shocks. Nothing feels right; they become disoriented and confused, and mourn their lost identity. Norm was one such fellow. He proudly described himself as having a "double Type A" personality: A legal shark whose prime directive was to swim forward and find money. For the four decades between receiving his Yale law degree and retirement from the firm he cofounded, Norm averaged 60-hour weeks and couldn't recall a sick day. After considerable coaxing and multiple postponements, he would begrudgingly go on vacations with his family, but always with a briefcase full of work. As technology improved, he proudly told me he was able to get as much done on safari in Kenya as he did at his Los Angeles office. "I'm bad, aren't I?" he asked with feigned shame and a wry smile. By working on vacation, he felt that he had eluded his wife's attempts to control him.

Going into retirement cold turkey caught him by surprise. He had earned it but had no idea what to do with it. His career had left no time for hobbies, sports, or friends, so there was nothing and no one waiting in the wings. He spent his first weeks of retirement drinking lunch and sleeping through the afternoon. This pattern left him sleepless most nights, alone with his thoughts, and not liking his own company. He began to realize that he didn't know his children and that they had grown up and established their lives in other cities without him. All his friends were at the firm, still working his old schedule and never available to get together. When he visited the office, everyone was glad to see him—as they passed him in the hall running to their next meeting. He became envious of his former colleagues and began to strategize about how to "unretire."

Norm was referred for psychotherapy by his internist, who had given him medication for insomnia and depression. He avoided calling me for months, until the day his wife asked him to do the dishes. When Norm found himself standing at the sink crying, he decided to give me a call. A week later, Norm sat across from me and asked, "What is happening to me? I don't understand why I'm such a mess." It was obvious that he was a man accustomed to getting down to business. His sentences shot out in rapid succession. "It must relate to leaving the firm because I was fine until I stopped working. I lie awake at night thinking of excuses to go back to work. I've even thought about moving to another city and starting a new firm. The crazy thing is, I have more money than I could ever spend and I've got a wonderful family—we're even expecting our first grandchild in a couple of months. What is happening to me?" The more he spoke, the more desperate he seemed to become. His state of mind was contagious, and I could feel myself getting increasingly agitated.

As I took in his experience, he continued, "My wife asked me to do the dishes, and it made me cry. Can you believe it—a grown man washing dishes and crying like a baby? What am I crying about? Everything is fine—we're healthy, we live in a huge house, we have good neighbors, complete freedom, we can buy anything we want, do anything we want to do—we have all the time in the world. Why do I feel like I'm going to jump out of my skin?" Norm looked me straight in the eye, pointed his two index fingers at me, and said, "Okay. GO!" Caught up in Norm's exploding emotions, I had forgotten about having to respond.

It appeared obvious that Norm's brain had been shaped to separate his conscious awareness and his inner experience. His ability to suppress his feelings had served him well in surviving a difficult childhood, serving in the military, and fighting the daily battle of courtroom litigation. I imagined that neural networks dedicated to thinking and feeling biased toward the left and right hemispheres had developed with insufficient cross talk and functional integration. His brain appeared to have been shaped in this fashion through a combination of temperament and experience. The challenge now was to resculpt it in a way that would allow him to adapt to new challenges.

Although Norm's image of himself was that of a fearless soldier, it was painfully obvious that he was ill equipped for life during peacetime. I knew that he was not ready to deal with his feelings directly. He needed a way of thinking about what was happening that would allow him to approach his internal world slowly while maintaining his pride. Norm needed a new story about himself and the meaning of his life, and a plan to guide him into the future. So instead of responding directly to his command, I began by telling him a story.

"While you were talking, I was reminded of a veteran I worked with some years ago. He went to Vietnam in his early 20s and did three tours of duty before coming home. He was highly decorated, loved the men in his platoon, and would have signed up for a fourth tour if the war hadn't ended. He came to therapy 15 years after the war because he was still having a hell of a time adjusting to being home. He had a great wife and two children he adored, but he was always anxious and afraid. He stayed up most nights and walked the perimeter of his property like he was on guard duty. Planes and helicopters going overhead or cars backfiring would have him diving for cover. What we've learned over the past decades is that brains adapt to crisis and often need help readjusting after the crisis has past. So while you and I know that this situation isn't a matter of life and death, the primitive parts of your brain may not understand the difference."

Norm identified with this experience, as it seemed to capture his imagination. He had no problem seeing himself as a combat veteran who needed to adjust to civilian life. He shared some recent experiences of being startled out of sleep in a cold sweat because he had dreamed that he missed a filing deadline or went into court unprepared for an important case. These discussions slowly led us to explore the typical architecture of the male brain, its biases, and the adaptational challenges men face in middle and later adulthood.

Always up for a challenge, once Norm had a map of the territory, he engaged in therapy with his usual focus and energy. I constantly encouraged him to be aware of how he was feeling along the way and mindful of the choices he was making throughout the day. This wasn't easy for him, and I had to find many ways to help him be more aware of his body, discover sensations, and attach them to conscious emotions. But by the time his first grandchild arrived, he had taken the first steps on the long path to becoming a more centered and emotionally available elder, preparing him to contribute to his family in a new way.

Part
Three

ATTACHMENT
AND WISDOM

7

The Emergence of Wisdom and Compassion

No wise man ever wished to be younger.
—Jonathan Swift

Now THAT WE HAVE EXPLORED THE INEXTRICABLE relationship between the vitality of our brains and our continued social embeddedness, we turn to what could be considered humanity's greatest achievements—wisdom and compassion. Traditionally associated with advanced age, wisdom and compassion are undoubtedly related to building and maintaining a healthy brain. Over the next four chapters, we will explore the emergence of wisdom and compassion in order to deepen our understanding of the purpose of our social brains.

To make the quantum leap from knowledge to wisdom, many interdependent accomplishments need to fall into place. Socially, we need to stay attached to those around us in meaningful ways. We need to be respected by and contribute to our community so as to enhance our sense of responsibility and belonging. Psychologically, we have to continue to learn, accept our aging and mortality, and embrace our role as elders. We have to cherish our storehouse of memories and experiences and pass them on to the next generation. Finally, wise elders need brains that support empathic attunement, careful consideration of complex social situations, and deepening compassion. The sustained activity of our attachment networks, a tendency to be less anxious and fearful, and our increasing abilities to solve complex social problems interact to make the emergence of wisdom possible.

The developmental course of the brain points us toward the attainment of wisdom as the elders' time-honored contribution to the tribe. Because the mind and the brain from which it arises are simultaneously embedded within biological, psychological, and social processes, maturational changes must occur at all three levels in order for wisdom to emerge. Given that wisdom goes back into our deep history, it is perhaps best seen in the fables, fairytales, and stories that have carried across the generations from time immemorial.

LIFE ON THE MISSISSIPPI

What wisdom can you find that is greater than kindness?
                                        Jean-Jacques Rousseau

History shows us that wisdom is a dish made up of many ingredients including experience, exposure to new people, and being open to ideas different from our own. We find a wonderful example of the awakening of wisdom in one of Mark Twain's most famous works. From a distance, *Huckleberry Finn* is a story of America's coming of age; a tale of two runaways, a white boy, Huck, and an escaped slave named Jim, rafting down the Mississippi.

Consistent with 19th-century American dogma, Huck had been taught that people of African descent were not wholly human and that slavery was condoned and encouraged by God. Being closer to farm stock than people, slaves needed the white man's care and direction in order to survive and live lives of purpose. In fact, having to take care of their slaves was considered just another aspect of the "white man's burden." Assured that slaves were indifferent to their families, he learned that they could be easily separated when bought and sold and gladly acquiesced to their masters' wishes.

Given these beliefs, you can imagine Huck's confusion when he heard Jim crying for his wife and family, lamenting that he was not there to love and protect them. He was surprised to find that Jim wanted no part of a master and clung to his freedom, pledging to work hard, save money, and buy back his family. He vowed that if their master wouldn't sell them, he would find an abolitionist and steal them. At first Huck was horrified—Jim was talking about stealing someone else's property! Further, in aiding a runaway slave, Huck was himself committing a crime against God. He could be sent to jail and, surely worse, go to hell.

Huck was at a crossroads. On one side stood everything he had ever been taught justifying slavery and the superiority of the white race. On the other were his experiences with Jim, a devoted friend, father, and husband; a fully human being. Huck's assumptions were turned upside down, throwing him into a state of turmoil. At one point, Huck's old ways of thinking gained the upper hand when he became convinced that he had committed a terrible sin in helping Jim to escape. Driven by guilt and the need to repent, he wrote a letter to Jim's owner to let her know where her property could be found. As he set the completed letter down on the table before him, he felt a sense of relief and marveled at how close he had come to eternal damnation. But then he reflected:

> I see Jim before me all the time: in the day and in the night-time, sometimes moonlight, sometimes storms, and we a-floating along, talking and singing and laughing. But somehow I couldn't seem to strike no places to harden me against him, but only the other kind. I'd see him standing my watch on top of his'n, 'stead of calling me, so I could go on sleeping . . . and do everything he could think of for me . . . and said I was the best friend old Jim ever had in the world, and the only one he's got now; and then I happened to look around and see that paper.
>
> . . . I took it up, and held it in my hand. I was a-trembling, because I'd got to decide, forever, betwixt two things, and I knowed it. I studied a minute, sort of holding my breath,

and then says to myself: "All right, then, I'll go to hell"—
and tore it up.[1]

Huck's choice is a well-known and much-loved expression of wisdom and compassion. But such profound wisdom from a young boy? Well, not quite. We know that behind Huckleberry Finn was the psyche and soul of an intelligent, introspective, and worldly Mark Twain. Huck's words and wisdom were born of Twain's extensive experience with the exciting and troubling admixture of realities that gave birth to the social experiment called the United States. Over a century later, we still find ourselves on that same raft.

WHAT IS WISDOM?

There is a wisdom of the head, and a wisdom of the heart.

Charles Dickens

Although we know it when we see it, wisdom defies easy definition. In fact, each chapter of a book about wisdom, edited by Yale psychologist Robert Sternberg, puts forth a somewhat different definition.[2] In the East, wisdom has traditionally focused on understanding and controlling one's thoughts and passions, as well as the ability to promote social harmony.[3] In Western cultures, wisdom appears as good advice, codes of social behavior, and an understanding of the meaning of life. In recent centuries, Western ideas of wisdom have taken a rational turn, coming to be more closely associated with knowledge. After a century of contact, Eastern and Western notions of wisdom are blending to create a view of wisdom as an embodiment of one's knowledge and compassion expressed in the context of relationships.[4]

We tend to think of wisdom as simultaneously grounded in a deep subjective experience of our emotional self and in an abiding awareness of our common humanity. In essence, wisdom is the result of an "inclusive way of experiencing the world," a combination of self and other in what Dan Siegel calls the "mind."[5] And while knowledge gives you the capacity to understand what you are doing, wisdom helps you to attain a just application of that knowledge. This is probably why knowledge can be judged against objective standards while wisdom is recognized in the heart and through group consensus.[6]

Who comes to mind when you think of a wise person? Someone from your childhood who made an impression on you? A philosopher, minister, or guru? When a group of undergraduates were asked to name well-known wise individuals, their top ten choices were as follows:[7]

1. Gandhi
2. Confucius
3. Jesus
4. Martin Luther King Jr.
5. Socrates
6. Mother Teresa
7. Solomon
8. Buddha
9. The Pope
10. Oprah Winfrey

This list contains an interesting mix of people, cultures, and historical eras. You may notice that we don't see Napoleon or Madam Curie on this list, so power and intellect aren't synonymous with wisdom. Similarly, we don't see any presidents, generals, or Wall Street tycoons. Instead, those who are thought of as wise are known more for their insight, compassion, and courage. In fact, four of the first five died because of their beliefs. In looking over this list, you may have an emotional reaction to one or more of these people. I certainly have one when I think back to the speeches of Dr. King that I heard as a young man. Perhaps this kind of emotional reaction to other human beings, the neural networks they stimulate, and the biochemical processes they trigger are aspects of how we identify wisdom—a sense that comes from the heart and gut as well as the brain.

With these thoughts in mind, I asked a group of graduate students to list the qualities they felt made someone wise. They were quick to point out that wisdom brings together both intellectual and emotional intelligence in ways that focus on our common humanity. The consensus was that wisdom emerges in the context of people coming together to comprehend and solve important social problems. I jotted down some of what they said and sorted their descriptions into three categories: a broad perspective, personal attributes, and attitudes toward others. See Table 7.1 for some of the descriptors of wisdom that emerged from our discussions.

Table 7.1. Aspects of Wisdom

A Broad Perspective

Self-awareness/Knowing what is important/Getting down to essentials

Seeing the bigger picture/Rising above one's own personal needs and cultural traditions

Understanding that knowledge is fallible/Maintaining a balance of knowledge and doubt

Personal Attributes

Moral principles and the courage to stand by them

Achieving a certain amount of detachment and not getting caught up in the moment

Ability to handle difficult situations well

Attitudes Toward Others

Empathic/Caring/Concerned/Forgiving

Being kind, loving, and compassionate

Understanding and accepting that people are fallible

According to this small and informal survey, attaining wisdom involves being able to see past the surface issues to deeper levels of meaning. Wise individuals are also able to discard notions of a singular correct perspective and remain open to new learning while recognizing limitations and distortions in their own thinking. A good example of this attitude comes from Michelangelo, who, in his ninth decade of life, wrote above his studio door, *Ancora Imparo* (I'm still learning); it is such a simple statement of insight and humility from the creator of *David* and the ceiling of the Sistine Chapel.

Research suggests that wisdom coalesces from a complex pattern of personality variables, life experience, and inner growth.[8] Those judged as wise in any age group excel in coping with existential issues and grasp the relativism of values.[9] They tend to have a rich internal life, good social skills, and remain open to new experiences.[10] People with wisdom are capable of sustaining their focus on a problem, consider its multiple dimensions and their personal responsibility in the matter.[11] Given that navigating complex and difficult relationships is one of life's most enduring challenges, much of wisdom is expressed in how people interact with and treat one another. Looking back to our list of wise people, most could be considered social revolutionaries who attempted to uplift the oppressed and/or serve the common good.

THE MATURATION OF THOUGHT

One has only to grow old to become more tolerant. I see no fault that I might not have committed myself.

Goethe

Is there anything about the maturation of thought that points toward the emergence of wisdom? And is there any relationship between how we think and whether we become wise? Piaget's stages of cognitive development unfold as a consequence of normal brain development. The progression from concrete to abstract thinking he describes follows a predictable course as cortical and subcortical neural networks mature and integrate. Wisdom, on the other hand, appears not to be a natural consequence of aging but a quantum leap from the linear unfolding of intellectual and emotional intelligence. But can we find any clues?

For adolescents and young adults, problem solving means gathering information quickly, presenting your argument, and convincing others you are right. A final solution is sought as soon as possible based on the available information and, once accepted, is energetically defended. All of these tendencies are manifestations of the reflexive search for means-end connections generated by immature brains. Younger people, I remember all too well, tend to assume the existence of a single valid answer and do not commonly come to new ways of thinking through disagreement and discussion. Table 7.2 contains a list of factors typically found in the problem-solving strategies of less mature thinkers.

The way adolescents and young adults think about problems may be tied to their primary developmental challenge— appearing competent and constructing an impressive social identity. A central component in this process involves creating an idealized identity. As the young person is confronted with new and more attractive options, each one is tried on and, for a time, feels like the final and best one. As part of their search for absolute truths, adolescents and young adults hold themselves and others to high standards tied to abstract ideals. Many use their identification with these ideals to avoid the anxiety of uncertainty and place responsibility for problems on others. This must sound familiar to those with adolescent children or with good memories.

Table 7.2. Characteristics of Immature and Mature Thinkers[a]

Less Mature Thinkers	More Mature Thinkers
A need for certainty and control	Tolerance of ignorance and lack of certainty
Limited recognition of complexity	Appreciation and acceptance of complexity
An inability to incorporate opposites	An ability to incorporate opposites
A lack of openness to unconscious processes	Openness to unconscious processes and influence
Belief that all important information is apparent	Tolerance for the time it takes to gather evidence
Lower empathic abilities	Greater empathy, sympathy and compassion
Less mature psychological defenses: denial, blame, and projection	More mature psychological defenses: humor, sublimation, and suppression

As thinking matures, it brings an increasing aware-ness of the complexity of human experience and the lim-its of human understanding. A reflexive response with obvious solutions gives way to slower deliberation and an awareness that not all of the relevant information may be immediately apparent. Most important, experience teaches us that solutions to human problems are hardly ever simple or straightforward. The accretion of experience provides a framework that allows us to sit with ambiguity while we ponder complex situations. This requires both the emotional regulation required to face the anxiety of uncertainty and an ability to remain patient while finding solutions. This kind of processing takes mature, integrated, and emotionally sophisticated brains. This is why older adults are better able to balance their views and self-interests with the needs and perspectives of others.[12]

It seems certain that the potential to become wise depends not only upon the accumulation of experience and intellectual abilities, but also upon positive emotional development. It is this emotional intelligence that allows us to maximize our intellect in the service of ourselves and others. As we will see in Chapter 8, evidence suggests that neurological changes related to aging may contribute to emotional regulation. Because emotions provide the platform for thought, emotional maturation is a necessary prerequisite for the quantum leap from thought to wisdom.

PSYCHOLOGICAL GROWTH

Knowledge speaks, but wisdom listens.
                    Jimi Hendrix

For almost a half century, ground zero of Western developmental theory has been the eight life stages of Erik Erikson. Erikson's model charted the psychological challenges that must be faced and overcome in order to be able to "love and work." Erikson's model extends from birth to young adulthood, with the eighth and final stage allocated to an undetermined period during later adulthood. In Table 7.3, you can see the names of Erikson's developmental stages on the left and what is accomplished if each stage is successfully navigated on the right.

Table 7.3. Erik Erikson's Developmental Stages[a]

1. Basic trust vs. basic mistrust	Infancy	Security/hope/optimism
2. Autonomy vs. shame	2 years	Self-esteem/emotional regulation
3. Initiative vs. guilt	4 years	Build skills/cooperate with others
4. Industry vs. inferiority	6 years+	Mastery of formal life skills
5. Identity vs. identity diffusion	13 years+	Certainty/self-confidence
6. Intimacy vs. isolation	Young adult	Friendships/enduring loves
7. Generativity vs. self-absorption	Young adult	Love/work
8. Integrity vs. despair	Later adulthood	The accumulated result of the first seven stages

The progression of psychological challenges described by Erikson contains the gradual creation of personal identity. The first two challenges occur in the context of early life within the home, while stages 3 through 5 are played out in school and peer relationships. Stages 6 and 7 are the hurdles reflected in establishing a family, intimate relationships, and a career, while stage 8 is a state of mind resulting from the successful navigation of the first seven. This model is heavily weighted toward early childhood while growing increasingly vague in adulthood: seven stages dedicated to the first third of life and one stage for the last two-thirds. The enormous status of childhood and the obvious bias of Erikson's model highlight the traditional lack of focus on adult development in Western psychology.

George Vaillant, a student of Erikson, has followed groups of men throughout their lives, interviewing them at multiyear intervals searching for correlates of healthy and unhealthy aging. He witnessed firsthand their increasing concern for others, the accumulation of wisdom, and the importance of communicating what they had learned to the next generation. Based on Erikson's model, it would be expected that these concerns would be minimal early in life, peak in midlife, and decline with increasing age. Contrary to this belief and in line with our present thesis, generativity concerns remain important throughout life and, in many ways, grow stronger with age.[13]

Vaillant also saw the importance of coming to a personal understanding of the meaning of one's life experiences. Based on his research, Vaillant reformulated Erikson's stages with a much-needed balance of focus on developmental stages across the life span and an emphasis on the passing on of knowledge and tradition (Table 7.4). The last three stages—generativity, keeper of the meaning, and integrity—are consistent with the traditional roles of elders around the world. Compare Vaillant's stages and his descriptions to those of Erikson.

Table 7.4. Vaillant's Reformulation of Erikson's Stages[a]

1. Identity: a sense of self distinct from one's parents
2. Intimacy: the development of reciprocal relationships
3. Career consolidation: finding a task that is valuable to self and society
4. Generativity: care for the next generation
5. Keeper of the meaning: passing on the traditions of the past to the next generation
6. Integrity: achieving a sense of peace and unity with respect to one's life and the world

One of the many ideas to emerge from Freudian psychoanalysis was the concept of defenses. The primary role of defenses is to decrease anxiety by distorting how we experience the more challenging aspects of reality. Mature defenses, such as humor, help us to cope with anxiety, which supports reality testing and our ability to love and work. Immature defenses, such as avoidance, denial, and dissociation, distort our thinking and emotions and hinder the formation of healthy attachments and attunement to the subjective state of others. These types of defenses make compassion and wisdom almost impossible.

Vaillant found that the vast majority of his subjects demonstrated a maturing of defenses that allowed for better coping skills and a greater ability to nurture themselves and others. Vaillant stated, "Successful aging means giving to others joyously whenever one is able, receiving from others gracefully whenever one needs it, and being greedy enough to develop one's own self in between."[14] In this same tradition, take a look at Gene Cohen's list of developmental imperatives for the maturing mind (Table 7.5).

Table 7.5. Cohen's Developmental Imperatives for the Maturing Mind [a]

1. To finally get to know and be comfortable with oneself

2. To learn how to live well

3. To have good judgment

4. To feel whole—psychologically, interpersonally, spiritually— despite loss and pain

5. To live life to the fullest right to the end

6. To give to others, one's family, and community

7. To tell one's story

8. To continue the process of discovery and change

9. To remain hopeful despite adversity

Although Valliant and Cohen don't mention wisdom explicitly, notice the overlap between the maturational processes this describe and the descriptions of wisdom earlier in this chapter. Wisdom is an expression of inner growth and interpersonal generativity based on cognitive and emotional maturation.

WISE ELDERS

Wisdom is a sacred communion.

Victor Hugo

While age is usually associated with wisdom, we see that age sometimes shows up all by itself. Age is associated with wisdom only for those with higher levels of emotional development, moral reasoning, and investment in other people.[15] Wise elders have spent a lifetime preparing for this role. They came to serve as the glue for their families and communities and are sought out for their knowledge, guidance, and comfort. Wise elders will likely be those individuals who stay mentally and physically vital throughout life.[16] Furthermore, since wisdom reflects an integration of brain functioning, it should also correlate with better physical and mental health, mature psychological defenses, and life satisfaction.[17] What is most striking is that so many older adults care so deeply for those around them, feel the urge to nurture, teach, and mentor others, and are vitalized by giving of themselves.

Wisdom emerges from and is expressed within relationships. Wise elders often have strong support systems and the respect of their community.[18] I would risk speculating that the same neurobiological principles at work with young children are also present in older adults. That is, being adored and appreciated helps to stimulate brain growth and supports health. People seeking our advice may stimulate our brains in ways that serve to make us more reflective, responsible, and caring.

Many years ago, I spent time on a reservation in southern Arizona and had the opportunity to speak to a number of Native Americans considered to be tribal elders. Sitting beneath a tree one blisteringly hot afternoon, I had the opportunity to talk with a man called Mister John. His bright eyes were sunken deep within a patchwork of dark wrinkles, and although he did not know his own age, I estimated him to be about 80 years old. I asked him about wisdom, and here, to the best of my recollection, is some of what he told me.

Back when I was a child, our people had no books, no television, and no radio. At night my grandfather would tell stories of a time before the white men, before the present constellations, back to the beginnings of our people. These stories connected us to our ancestors and before them to the gods, and before that to the earth. His stories were considered a sacred lifeline to our history, and my grandfather was a vessel of these stories. As links in this chain, everyone in the tribe was important, especially the old ones, who would have answers to questions in difficult times. As these stories collected within me, I felt fuller, richer, and safer on the earth.

He told me that as he was growing up, the young men of the tribe would get into fights, and that on occasion feuds between families would erupt. In these situations, the tribal elders functioned as peacekeepers who, through their stories and counsel, would try to give each party a different way of seeing the conflict. They would remind the feuding families that peace was more important than winning an argument because as a tribe, the fates of all were interwoven. They taught the tribe that when people are fighting, the only path to resolution is seeing the situation through the eyes of your enemy.

The old man cleared his throat and continued:

The main problem I see in the white man's culture is that the adults look to their children for answers while the elders are ignored and put in old folks' homes. How will the children learn who they are? Children don't know how to act without being shown. Children are sponges that absorb whatever touches them. If all they see is television and movies, they will behave like bandits and cartoon animals.

People have a feeling of having lost something very important, but have no idea of what it might be. I think it is connection. People need families and families need tribes. If the family is not a part of a tribe, children will naturally go out seeking a tribe. Fortunate children find sports teams or hobbies they can share with friends. The unlucky ones find gangs or go into the army and get killed. They are seeking their tribe, but there is no tribe like your real tribe.

This lack of a tribe also hurts the old ones. The elders need to see younger ones looking at them who are hungry for their stories. Without younger listeners, old ones get confused and lose their memories. They become sad and lost and wither away. We all need a connection with our past through our ancestors, down into the earth. These connections have been lost to the white man and even many of my own people. Without our ancestors, we may become forever lost and wander the earth.

I've tried to teach my children and grandchildren that wisdom is earned over a lifetime. Each day, you must do something that strengthens your spirit and deepens your wisdom. This is how, when you become old, you will have value to your tribe. This is your retirement plan. Right from the beginning of life, guide your thoughts, pick your friends, and choose your words wisely. Think of how to become a benefit to yourself and others when you are an old one. Make yourself a tree heavy with fruit and you will always find others gathered around you. These people will be your life's riches.

Mister John could have filled many books with his wisdom.

8

The Maturation of Emotion

*When the passions relax their hold, then you
have escaped from the control not of one master,
but of many.*

—Plato

Y OU MAY HAVE NOTICED THAT IT IS DIFFICULT TO
be compassionate or wise when you feel anxious, afraid, or
stressed. In fact, when we feel that we are under threat, our
cortex becomes inhibited and brain processing shifts to networks that specialize in immediate survival and away from
measured judgment, self-awareness, and a broad perspective. This doesn't happen only when we are chased by wild
animals; the same brain shift occurs in our day-to-day lives
when we are hungry, angry, lonely, tired, or in any state of
emotional dysregulation. This shift from cortical to subcortical brain processing is one of the major causes of difficulties in raising children, maintaining marriages, and success
at work.

The ability to stay mindful of both our social roles and our internal emotional state supports compassion and wisdom. It also enhances neural plasticity, integration, and brain health. Anxious families demand obedience and loyalty to the family rules, no matter how destructive they might be for one and all. The same is true for fragile totalitarian regimes and businesses with insecure CEOs. The more afraid we become, the more likely we are to resort to rigid ideologies, behaviors, and policies.

LEARNING NOT TO FEAR

The human brain starts working the moment you are born and never stops until you stand up to speak in public.

George Jessel

In thinking about how changes in the maturing brain are conducive to wisdom, we return our focus to two brain regions, the amygdala and the orbitomedial prefrontal cortex (OMPFC). As we saw earlier, it is within the OMPFC-amygdala networks that our ability to regulate our emotions becomes organized. The amygdala is a primitive structure that rapidly scans for danger and, if necessary, mobilizes the body into action by activating the fight-flight response.[1] The OMPFC is capable of regulating and inhibiting the amygdala when an extreme emotional response is unnecessary or counterproductive. When the OMPFC is damaged in some way, we become more vulnerable to depression, mania, and antisocial behavior.[2]

Together, the OMPFC and the amygdala remember the value of social interactions from early attachment to the day we die.[3] On its own, the amygdala is capable of unconsciously processing interactions of which we are totally unaware, making us automatically react to and avoid people, places, and things that have previously had a negative effect on us.[4] These capabilities lead the amygdala to have a very important role in both our conscious and unconscious experience. Even if we try our best to be mindful of our moment-to-moment emotional experience, the amygdala can shape our thoughts, feelings, and behaviors before conscious awareness.[5]

Because the OMPFC and the amygdala have a mutually inhibitory relationship, damage to the OMPFC results in less control over our behaviors, perceptions, and judgments.[6] In these situations, our thinking is guided less by conscious consideration and more by aggressive, authoritarian, and prejudicial impulses. We are also more likely to engage in compulsive and self-destructive behaviors such as substance abuse, binge eating, or lashing out at others. On the other hand, when we are able to regulate our emotions, we optimize judgment and decision making. A highly developed and well-regulated OMPFC-amygdala network is a prerequisite for psychological maturity and the attainment of wisdom.

THE AMYGDALA NEVER FORGETS

Time moves in one direction, memory in another.

William Gibson

Why is it so easy to forget the name of someone you just met, but so hard to forget a traumatic experience? One reason lies in the differences between the hippocampus and amygdala. The hippocampus, central to explicit memory, remains flexible to new learning and even changes size with changing memory demands.[7] In contrast, the amygdala is like the proverbial elephant that never forgets bad experiences.[8] So while the hippocampus is constantly remodeling to keep abreast of current environmental changes, the amygdala catalogues past threats and rapidly applies them to new experiences.

Unlike our fragile memories for names and dates, the amygdala has a tenacious memory for what has frightened us. Adding to the tenacity of trauma is the fact that amygdala activation results in chemical processes that actually enhance memories for bad experiences. In scientific terms, our fears are resistant to extinction because natural selection has shaped them this way to protect us from similar threats in the future.

The only brain structure whose size is positively correlated with longevity in primates is the central portion of the amygdala.[9] Might a larger amygdala enhance survival and be chosen by natural selection? As primates grow larger, they also live in larger and more complex social groups, creating the need for intricate social communication and vast memory stores for all of the interactions we have with others. Unfortunately for us, a large amygdala may also make us more vulnerable to social anxieties and phobias of all kinds.[10]

The establishment of secure attachments and positive affect regulation early in life allows us to regulate amygdala functioning as opposed to being victimized by the anxiety and fear it can activate. When a child is neglected or abused, his or her amygdala can become biased toward fear activation, which can emotionally cripple the individual in ways that can last a lifetime. Like a wild horse, the amygdala needs to be tamed to enhance its positive characteristics. With the amygdala, as with horses, taming occurs in the context of an understanding relationship—the establishment of control and regulation through a combination of affection and limit setting. When we share our wisdom and offer compassion to others, we are serving as amygdala whisperers to those whom we touch.

AMYGDALA WHISPERING

Life shrinks or expands in proportion to one's courage.

Anaïs Nin

For most of our lives, negative emotions weigh more heavily than positive ones in our evaluation of ourselves and others.[11] While it is generally assumed that aging results in an increase in fearfulness, the research shows an actual decrease of fear and anxiety with age.[12] Sixty- to 80-year-olds show decreased amygdala activity and increased frontal lobe activation while analyzing facial expressions.[13] These changes are not due to a decline of amygdala functioning but to a change in the OMPFC-amygdala balance toward decreased fear processing.[14] In line with this finding, older individuals also show less cardiovascular reactivity (triggered by amygdala activation) when watching emotionally charged films.[15] Thus, there appears to be an age-related shift away from anxiety that may be an important contributor to the emergence of compassion and wisdom.

It has been found that as we age, we are influenced less by the way questions are framed when presented to us.[16] In other words, we are less likely to be influenced by the current situation or persuasion by others. The advantages of a less reactive amygdala are not just a relaxation of fear and anxiety, but increased cortical involvement allowing for slower and deeper reflection. The maturation of the OMPFC-amygdala circuit works against the impulses and mandates of youth to be certain and act fast.

In comparison to adolescents, older adults rely more on problem-focused than emotion-based reactions in difficult situations.[17] Advancing wisdom includes the expansion of consideration and taking time to understand the complexities of a situation. The general downgrading of fear later in life may open us to a deeper understanding and compassion for others, and more love for humanity in general. To a great degree, the experience of love is the absence of fear. The taming of the amygdala may be one of the primary gifts of aging and a component of becoming a more loving person.

ACCENTUATE THE POSITIVE

Wisdom begins in wonder.

Socrates

The OMPFC-amygdala network is so central to our social and emotional experience that any changes in its functioning are reflected across the board in memory, thinking, and personality. Research has shown that, far from being cranky and pessimistic, older individuals tend to retain positive emotions, while negative ones are more likely to decrease.[18] In general, older adults exhibit more emotional control and have fewer negative experiences.[19] This shift toward positivity with age has been found to occur from 18 to 60 years of age, at which point it seems to level off.[20]

As we age, research has shown that we tend to remember more positive and neutral visual images than negative ones.[21] Older subjects also tend to look away from faces with negative expressions and toward those with positive ones.[22] This likely relates to a decrease in the amygdala's guidance of the visual system, which emphasizes vigilance to negative and dangerous aspects of the environment.[23] Another study showed that when we look at faces with different emotions, we have greater activation in brain areas that reflect positive emotions as we age.[24]

Older subjects have also been found to have a greater bias toward remembering positive words than younger subjects, reflecting the OMPFC-amygdala system shift away from anxiety.[25] Overall, older adults tend to (1) experience fewer negative emotions, (2) pay less attention to negative stimuli, and (3) be less likely to remember negative experiences.[26] Older adults also show this positivity effect in recalling autobiographical memory and tend to spin their histories in ways that make them look more competent and feel better about themselves.[27]

This reminds me of the clothing brand Old Guys Rule, whose motto is "the older we get, the better we were." In this way, older adults probably don't differ from the rest of the population. However, when older adults are informed about the need for accuracy of recollection, this positivity bias diminishes, while younger subjects tend to hold onto their egocentric distortions. As we get older, we tend to show less emotional fluctuation, greater emotional regulation, and more understanding of our emotions. We're also better able to employ coping strategies when strong emotions arise.

The positivity effect on remembering and recounting life history edits our life story with a positive spin. The optimism this may engender correlates with enhanced physical and mental health.[28] It may also serve to instill hope in younger people, who have traditionally depended upon the stories of the elders to create a vision of the future. What better gift can we give to our children and grandchildren than grandparents who enjoy life and show them that despite hardships, life is very much worth living?

THE CYCLE OF OPTIMISM

Old people don't get crabby, crabby people get old.

Steve Otto

Optimism and a positive attitude correlate with physical and mental health, happiness, and longevity. Optimistic people are better connected, employ better coping skills, and take better care of themselves than pessimistic people. Pessimism earlier has been shown to be a risk factor for poor physical and mental health.[29] It has been shown that optimistic people are significantly less likely to be rehospitalized after bypass surgery, demonstrate quicker recovery patterns, and tend to have better survival rates after being diagnosed with head and neck cancer.[30]

In one study of patients with breast cancer, optimists were more likely to use coping mechanisms such as acceptance, humor, positive reframing, religion, and social support.[31] Optimistic beliefs about one's health predicted greater attention to medical information, better coping with bad news, and better emotional regulation while pursuing health care.[32] Optimistic people may have more positive expectations for success, so they approach difficult situations, expend energy to solve problems, and experience better outcomes.

If optimism enhances our emotional state and decreases stress, then it should also have a positive impact on our immunological functioning. In fact, an optimistic outlook has been associated with higher T-cell and natural killer cell levels in a healthy population, as well as slowed disease progression and lower mortality in patients with HIV.[33] This positive association among optimism and bodily health may explain why optimistic men have a slower progression of heart disease and are less likely to develop it in the first place.[34]

Considerable evidence suggests that optimism may be correlated with longevity.[35] In the United States, it was found that people who interpret events in pessimistic ways are more likely to become depressed, become physically ill, and die earlier.[36] Interestingly, a study of the oldest old in Veneto, Italy, found that centenarians were less inclined to complain about their physical condition and had a positive attitude toward life despite any disabilities.[37] Having a reason for living, a zest for life, and plans for the future went along with decreased mortality rates and better health 10 years later.[38] This is why it's always good to have a long-term project on your to-do list.

Seligman suggests that pessimism may increase mortality because pessimists (1) have more negative life events, (2) believe nothing they do makes a difference, or (3) have depressed immune systems.[39] Pessimism and hopelessness are also characteristics of depression, which has been shown to correlate with higher rates of mortality.[40] In one study of 5,201 people aged 65 years and older, the risk of mortality was

43% higher among individuals with depressive symptoms, while another study found depressive symptoms in women to be a significant risk factor for illness-related mortality.[41]

One explanation for this relationship may lie in differences in health behavior. Optimistic people tend to use proactive coping strategies that aim to eliminate, reduce, or manage stress and negative emotions.[42] Whether optimism is a cause of these positive outcomes or a natural consequence of robust health and living a good life is difficult to sort out.[43] It is safe to assume that optimism, social support, physical health, and longevity have positive synergistic effects on both well-being and longevity.

SHATTERED ASSUMPTIONS

The wound is the place where the light enters you.

Rumi

Although the reality of our mortality is present throughout life, optimism, denial, and other defenses help us to be oblivious to them most of the time. As we grow older, however, we start to gain an increasing recognition of the inevitability of death. The lucky ones among us have the luxury of confronting these existential realities gradually and in small doses. For many, suffering and loss come too hard and too early in life. When children and adolescents are traumatized, their assumptions of safety can be shattered, catapulting them into lifelong anxiety.

In stark contrast, traumatic experiences are also capable of enhancing self-discovery and supporting the attainment of compassion and wisdom. Think back for a moment to the list of the 10 wisest people:

1. Gandhi
2. Confucius
3. Jesus
4. Martin Luther King Jr.
5. Socrates

6. Mother Teresa
7. Solomon
8. Buddha
9. The Pope
10. Oprah Winfrey

Suffering played a role in the lives of many of these people, not just personal suffering, but shared suffering through their empathic attunement to the pain of others. Most of these wise people were transformed by their experiences and were motivated to act on behalf of others. They were, in a sense, able to regain control over their fear and shift back to cortical control. So while none of us would choose to suffer, the experience of suffering can play a central role in our personal histories. In fact, the central tenets of Buddhism are based on the belief that suffering is at the core of human existence and that transcendence of suffering is the path to enlightenment.

The most important aspect of early attachment relationships is the establishment of a sense of safety, which eventually gives us the strength to cope with life's more difficult realities. Because primates are such social animals, and our very survival depends on our connection with others, the more familiar, safe, and loving people there are in a child's life, the less likely she or he will feel alone, abandoned, or afraid. The maturation of brain systems that modulate fear and our ability to reframe life in a more positive manner are a valuable gift that elders can pass on to their children and grandchildren.

We have evolved from simple and separate biological organisms into conscious, social, and cultural creatures. In this long and complex evolutionary process, our experience of self and our sense of identity have expanded to include our families, friends, communities, and religious beliefs. We can now be traumatized, not only when our physical safety is at risk but when the people and ideals we care about are threatened.

NATHAN AND JOSHUA

Nathan and Joshua were father and son. Nathan, a hard-working and devout man, dedicated his life to taking care of his parents until he married in his 40s, and had Joshua, his only child. At 80, Nathan had "lost some spring from his step," but was quick to add he was "as sharp as a tack." Joshua was a caring, sensitive man and a gifted illustrator. Joshua and his father had always had a close and caring relationship that was grounded in deep love and mutual respect. Nathan was proud of his son's accomplishments, and Joshua was proud of his father.

For many years, Joshua secretly struggled with his sexual

identity and learned to skillfully deflect the usual questions from his parents about girlfriends, marriage, and a family. The year Joshua turned 37, he sat his parents down and told them he was gay. At first they sat frozen in stunned silence. After a few moments, his mother regained her equilibrium and told Joshua that she loved him. Nathan remained silent and eventually left the table without a word. Nathan's assumptions had been truly shattered, and he sank into an uncharacteristic depression. After a few weeks, he sought my help to try and make sense of what had happened.

"How could my son choose to be gay?" Nathan asked me during our first session. "He had a good home, never wanted for anything, went to the best schools. We gave him love, everything he asked for. . . . How could this happen?" I could see and feel the depths of Nathan's confusion, anger, and disappointment. "I've lost my son. How can I continue to have a relationship with him and expect one day to face God? It isn't possible. I can't believe I have to forsake my own son!" Nathan was indeed caught between a rock and a hard place. On one side stood a son whom he deeply loved and cherished, and on the other stood his beliefs, prejudices, and fears that had been shaped over a lifetime. There were so many conflicts running through his mind that I wasn't sure where to begin, so I just encouraged him to keep talking.

Over a number of sessions, Nathan told me about his early life, his marriage, and raising Joshua. Story after story poured forth, and I could see that he had done an excellent job of integrating the various aspects of his life into a coherent narrative. "I'm no Abraham," Nathan told me. "I can't sacrifice my son for my faith, yet I can't imagine living without my faith. I feel like I'm being torn in two." I was beginning to suspect that Nathan's all-or-nothing, black-and-white thinking was about to collapse. Here was an opening for me to move from a solely supportive position and become a collaborator in solving his dilemma. Thinking about it now, this would have been a good time for us to have read *Huckleberry Finn*.

We gathered information and read articles about homosexuality and how different religions have dealt with the issue. Nathan's thinking gradually shifted from assuming that homosexuality was a conscious choice to an appreciation of the power of biology on sexual identy and orientation. This shift in perspective went a long way in helping Nathan to see that his son was not doing this to hurt him or his family. We also read personal accounts of homosexual men, especially stories describing the anguish at coming out and being rejected by their parents. I shocked Nathan one day by reminding him that the extermination of homosexuals, along with the Jews, was part of Hitler's final solution. As he showed me pictures of Joshua as a young boy, he began to put the pieces together. He recalled Joshua's avoidance of sports, his lack of interest in girls, and how his room was always the best-decorated one in the house. He told me that when Joshua was 9, he had stopped his subscription to *Sports Illustrated* in preference for *Architectural Digest*.

"It's not easy to teach an old dog new tricks, is it, Lou?"

Nathan asked after many months of exploration and debate. "The truth is that I have no option but to love and accept my son. It's the right thing to do; it's the only thing I can do. If this is who he is, then I have to learn to understand and accept him. If it means that I have to change synagogues, rethink some of my beliefs, and deal with being embarrassed in front of my friends, so be it. He is my son, and nothing is more important." By now, both of us had tears in our eyes. Nathan had somehow found the strength, courage, and flexibility to deal with issues that required serious neural rewiring. This old dog had learned a new trick.

Nathan decided to invite Joshua to our next session because, as he said, "I might need some backup." The session was wonderful. Nathan began by apologizing for his recent distance, and Joshua quickly accepted his father's apology. He seemed to appreciate and respect what his father had been going through and had faith that he would eventually understand. Joshua talked about his struggle over the years with the dawning awareness of being gay and his fears about what it would mean to his family. Nathan looked over to me from time to time as Joshua described experiences similar to those we had read about. By the end of the session, Nathan asked Joshua to take it slow and give him a little time before he introduced him to his boyfriend. We all laughed.

In subsequent weeks, father and son spent time together and found a rabbi to speak to about their relationship. I was very impressed with Nathan and let him know it. During one of our final sessions, he recalled some of his experiences while serving in World War II. He told me that of all the lessons he learned, the most important was that life was confusing, beautiful, and fragile. "Nothing is more important than the people we love. If what I am doing is wrong," Nathan said, "I hope God can understand and forgive me."

Nathan had learned to regulate his emotions, face problems directly, and come to appreciate his own biases all the while keeping in mind what was truly important. In my eyes, Nathan was the embodiment of the deepest aspects of wisdom and the faith he lived by.

Challenges to Wisdom

*We are so thoroughly trained to follow our
thoughts that our mindfulness is weak.*

—Sakyong Mipham

So far we have seen that the attainment of
wisdom requires an ongoing integration of worldly experience, emotional maturation, self-awareness, and compassion.[1] This can be quite a challenge in the face of evolution's
other mandate to do unto others before they do unto us.
Wisdom and compassion sometimes requires a transcendence of personal well-being.

It is not a coincidence that throughout the world, wisdom is thought to go hand in hand with time spent in meditation, spiritual retreats, and religious pilgrimages. Time
spent apart from the moment-to-moment struggle for survival frees one to turn inward and explore the mechanisms
of mind and emotion. The more familiar we become with
the ways in which a human brain functions—its brilliant

achievements and profound shortcomings—the more likely we will be able to use our minds for higher purposes. Older people have a number of advantages when it comes to becoming wise. Their slower pace, broader perspective, and years of experience allow them to bring more information and perspective to any situation. Decreases in the distorting effects of fear and anxiety allow older individuals to see social situations with less defensiveness and more clarity. Because healthy maturing brains are characterized by widespread neural activation, they are better equipped to integrate emotion, intellect, and intuition.[2] Let's look at some of the ways in which healthy aging favors the emergence of wisdom.

SPEED VERSUS FLEXIBILITY

Age considers; youth ventures.

Rabindranath Tagore

One of the principles governing the evolution of complex neural systems is an optimal balance between response speed and response flexibility. Response speed is the time it takes us to successfully respond to a situation. Response flexibility is the number of appropriate options we are able to remember, consider, and choose from. Acting quickly requires a minimum of neural processing, while response flexibility requires slower analysis of more information and the use of more extensive brain regions. These two tendencies reflect the poles of our existence: On the one extreme, the most primitive reflexes of our brains' evolutionary past, and on the other, what it is able to accomplish with the trillions of newer neural connections.

Think about how quickly we pull our hand away from a hot stove or how we startle when touched from behind when we think we are alone. These rapid reactions have been hardwired through eons of natural selection. They occur so quickly that we can only consciously experience them in retrospect. An urban legend circulates through the greasy spoons of New York about a cook who saved his money for years to buy a very special watch. He polished it religiously each day and showed it off to everyone he met. One day as he was taking off his watch in his work kitchen, he accidentally dropped it into the fryer—reflexively, he reached into the boiling oil to retrieve it. This was not something he decided to do, but something he found was a bad idea only after realizing what he had done.

In fact, simple responses, such as the knee-jerk reflex that occurs when the doctor hits our knee with a rubber hammer, don't even reach our brains. They utilize a reflex arc involving the spinal cord. Basic fear responses don't require cortical involvement but are mediated via primitive subcortical structures (including the amygdala) to get our bodies immediately mobilized for fight or flight. The braking of a car during a panic stop is another good example, something that would simply take too long to process in the cortex.

If response speed is one side of the equation, the other

side is the cognitive, behavioral, and emotional flexibility that comes from assessing a situation, thinking through alternatives, and selecting what we feel to be the best option. During early development, we see a gradually increasing ability to inhibit impulses and bring past learning to bear during decision-making. As neural systems mature and integrate, they demonstrate increasingly sophisticated processing for more complex tasks. All of this occurs while simultaneously retaining the automatic reflexes that allow us to react to immediate threats.

As a rule of thumb, the more complex the analysis we engage in, the more widespread the neural participation and the more time it takes to respond. For example, when subjects are asked to make moral judgments in social situations, a wide array of cortical and subcortical regions become activated. Tasks requiring self-awareness, self-reflection, and empathy for others, recruit the involvement of broad social and cognitive neural networks.[3] The complex human problems that are the focus of wisdom call upon all of these networks in both cortical hemispheres as well as subcortical structures.

Subcortical activation reflects the involvement of networks that organize primitive drives and emotions, as we attune to and resonate with the participants caught up in whatever dilemma we are evaluating. Networks of the social brain become activated when we put ourselves in someone else's shoes. Finally, the prefrontal cortex contributes to our ability to process complex social interactions and

weigh potential outcomes. This wisdom is not an abandonment of primitive emotions, but an integration of deep
emotions that help us empathize with others and employ a
broader perspective.

Attention to internal feelings also adds valuable information for making social judgments. Younger people, fixed on
external information and environmental contingencies, are
less slowed by these mediating factors that are taken into
account by wise elders. In a study comparing young and old
subjects on a variety of tasks, the older adults (age 60–80),
while slower, performed as well or better, especially on tasks
requiring social judgment.[4] Older subjects have also been
found to be better at recalling their feelings about real and
imagined events than younger subjects.[5]

To act wisely, we have to simultaneously be aware of
our own biases, inhibit impulses that would make us act
rashly, and be empathic and caring toward others, all the
while applying our intellectual abilities to complex situations. In older age we can expect a reduction of processing
speed accompanied by an improvement in the pragmatics
of social problem solving.[6] Brain processing strategies that
make for quick decisions earlier in life seem to gradually give
way to the more inclusive and fine-tuned cerebral networks
required for wisdom.[7]

A senior pilot once told me that while younger pilots
react more quickly to emergency situations, more experienced pilots tend to avoid them in the first place. This
seems to be backed up by research with air traffic control-

lers. Although reaction time and memory are superior in 30-year-old air traffic controllers, those in their 60s do as well or better in simulated emergency situations. The combination of years of experience and changes in the brain results in the enhancement of complex skills over time. The emotional activation in high-pressure, high-stakes situations may also impair the cognitive functioning of younger pilots and controllers more than it does those with more experience and a tame amygdala. Listen to the tone of Captain Sullenberger's voice on the cockpit recorder after he was told to return to the airport, when he said, "We aren't going to make it; I'm putting her down on the Hudson."

BLAME VERSUS RESPONSIBILITY

A man can fail many times, but he isn't a failure until he begins to blame someone else.

John Burroughs

Through natural selection, our social brains evolved to quickly predict and react to the anticipated activities of others. Research in social neuroscience has demonstrated that we have a variety of neural systems dedicated to unconsciously monitoring the behavior of others that use body posture, gaze direction, facial expressions, and pupil dilation to predict behavior. These "mind-reading" systems are reflexive and fast, processing data far more quickly than the half second it takes for us to become consciously aware of what we are experiencing. They automatically generate an implicit theory of another's motivations, intentions, and likely behaviors. This theory of someone's state of mind provides us with both an early warning system for potential danger and a mechanism of interpersonal attunement and understanding.

While this kind of mind reading is automatic and instantaneous, we have no analogous system dedicated to self-awareness. In fact, some have proposed that self-awareness may be a disadvantage to survival because it slows down our reaction time and makes it more difficult to deceive ourselves and others. For example, if we are able to convince ourselves that we are innocent of a crime, we may be better able to fool others (and a lie detector) with our pleas of innocence. Using mind reading for deceptive purposes and personal gain is clearly demonstrated while playing poker, where the most consistent winners are those who are best at reading their opponents' "tells" while concealing their reactions behind a "poker face."

Many forms of self-deception appear to be baked into the human genome. For example, when others make a mistake, we tend to think that there is something wrong with their abilities, intelligence, or character. If, on the other hand, we make the same mistake, we tend to blame environmental factors—wind direction, fatigue, or the blunders of others that set us up to fail. This perceptual distortion, called the *fundamental attribution error*, shows that we are innately biased toward externalizing blame and looking to factors outside of ourselves for our own failures. A related phenomenon is what Freud called *projection*, a tendency to see our own faults in those around us while feeling free of blame ourselves. While attribution errors and projection are reflexive and serve to lessen anxiety and self-doubt, awareness of our own shortcomings requires effort and a willingness to tolerate negative feelings about ourselves.

All of us can spend hours describing the behaviors, motivations, and problems of other people and remain oblivious to the fact that we are actually describing ourselves. Couples are often completely convinced that the problems in the marriage are totally attributable to their spouses. I can relate to these states of mind because I often find myself doing the same thing. But blaming others is more than a character weakness; it is likely a natural consequence of the automatic mind-reading circuitry bequeathed to us from our evolutionary history. We automatically assess others but have no automatic process for assessing ourselves. This comes with the discipline and practice of self-reflection that is required if one is to become a truly wise person. In fact, wise individuals are mindful of these innate tendencies and learn to use their judgments of others as windows to the hidden corners of their own inner worlds.

Unfortunately, self-awareness, personal responsibility, and common sense are not that common—just watch the news or read a newspaper. The evolution of consciousness requires remembering who we are, deepening our appreciation of our interconnectedness, and learning how to listen and love rather than talk and blame. Placing our individual views in a social perspective, knowing our prejudices, and appreciating the importance of human relationships take dedication and effort. This kind of self-awareness, along with wisdom and compassion, may soon become a requirement for our continued survival as a species. As the world grows smaller, it is clear that we will need to evolve to a higher level of social consciousness.

REFLEX VERSUS REFLECTION

The art of being wise is the art of knowing what to overlook.

William James

Our brains have evolved to look outward and be on alert. When we are safe, our aggression may get channeled into exercise and sports; when food is readily available, our primitive drives to forage get converted into hobbies and home improvement projects. When reflexes and primitive drives get caught in the "on" position, we can develop all kinds of compulsive behaviors. Many of us spend time preoccupied with to-do lists or caught up in a never-ending chain of thoughts that keeps our minds spinning.

Jon had been my client for years and complained about having too many things to do. We examined his schedule, talked about cutting back on work and social obligations, and created lists of priorities from which he was to trim off the bottom third. Despite countless discussions and repeated repentance, Jon continued to be extremely over-committed. It eventually became clear that he had made coming to therapy another thing on his to-do list. Instead of using it to make his life better, Jon had unknowingly turned therapy into part of his problem.

In the process of exploring what kept Jon going so fast and furious, all roads led to anxiety and fear. He was afraid that if he didn't work every bit of available overtime, he would run out of money. If he didn't keep everything under control, "all hell would break loose." If he didn't do every-thing his friends asked him to do, he would end up unloved and alone. Despite seeing the irrationality of his behaviors, nothing changed. Jon was just too frightened to even experi-ment with slowing down.

Meanwhile, Jon's son was acting out in school, and his daughter was showing signs of depression. Jon's wife described herself as a single parent, and his children's thera-pist suggested that it might help if Jon spent more time with his family. Jon understood that his anxiety-driven behavior was damaging to him and his entire family, yet nothing I said—nothing anyone said—seemed to have an impact on his behavior. Just when I was beginning to think the situa-tion might be hopeless, Jon came into a session with a big smile and the following story:

> Last Wednesday morning, I was trimming my toenails before getting dressed. I got through the first nine and

was about to start cutting the tenth when the phone rang. It was a call from work, and I had to go to my desk to jot down some notes. I was running late, so I put on my socks and shoes and ran out the door without cutting the last toenail. For days I was aware of that toenail, feeling it snag on my sock when I got dressed in the morning, scratching the sheets at night before I passed out. Then I forgot about it. As I was driving here this morning I realized that a week had gone by and I still hadn't cut it. It was so long now that I could push it against the inside of my shoe. Suddenly it hit me—my wife and kids, even my own health are all tenth toenails. There's something about this toenail that made me realize I must be crazy. I think I'm ready to start therapy.

Jon's story highlights many important issues. The first is that compulsivity is self-reinforcing because it reduces anxiety. In Jon's case, his anxieties about his own worth were relieved by constantly doing for others. Anxiety is the enemy of behavioral flexibility, neural plasticity, and self-insight. When we feel anxious or afraid, we focus on acting on the environment, forgetting who we are and what is important to us. Because he felt that his wife and kids were already his, they required little of the fear-driven attention he showed others. For years this psychological dynamic remained invisible to Jon. It took the metaphor of an uncut toenail and his sense of humor to break the spell. Jon was lucky. For most people, it takes a life-threatening illness, a trip to the emergency room with a panic attack, or the loss of a loved one to wake up from the spell of compulsivity.

Getting to know ourselves involves turning attention away from the demands, expectations, and details of the external world, and turning inward. While behavior is more widely studied because it is readily observable and easily measured, our inner experience is just as important. Traditionally avoided by researchers, the subjective aspects of human experience are now receiving increasing attention as emotion, empathy, and the effects of meditation on the brain have become areas of interest for research and the popular press.

It is important to keep in mind that the frontal and parietal lobes initially evolved to allow us to navigate in space and across time. This frontal-parietal system has more recently given us the ability to navigate an internal world of imagination.[8] This inner space can serve as a safe, reflective context in which to detach from the demands of the outer world in order to self-reflect and engage in deep consideration.

A quiet and safe internal world, once created, can be revisited, providing a context for private thought separate from external problem solving. These quiet moments serve as the grounds for imagination and creativity and are especially important for children in the process of forming an experience of self.[9] One's conscious sense of self consolidates during times of still reflection and creates the possibility for greater empathy for others and ourselves.

The parietal lobes, located above our ears, are at the

crossroads of the neural networks responsible for vision, and hearing. They serve as a high-level association area for the integration and coordination of our senses and connect them with conscious thought.[10] During periods of contemplation and quiescence, there is a shift from frontal to parietal activation.[11] In fact, the same shift occurs when experienced meditators engage in meditation.[12]

Research has shown that greater amounts of gray matter in the temporal, parietal, and frontal lobes later in life are related to things like mature creativity, openness to divergent feelings and thoughts, and a sense of connectedness with others and the world.[13] In fact, the middle regions of the parietal lobes appear to be a hub of self-representation, memory of ourselves in the world, and reflective self-awareness.[14]

The fact that most professionals don't think of the parietal lobes as a component of the executive brain may reflect a cultural bias of equating individuals with their external behavior rather than their inner emotional experiences. Interestingly, studies of skulls reflecting different stages of primate evolution suggest that expansion of the parietal lobes is more characteristic of the human brain than expansion of the frontal lobes.[15] We have seen that as we age there appears to be greater neural loss in frontal than parietal regions. Could the neural loss we see with age somehow support the development of enhanced mindfulness?

Narcissism in its many forms can be understood as a failure to create a secure inner world. Instead they have to rely on external validation for a sense of emotional regulation and well-being. In many ways, narcissism is the opposite of both intellectual and emotional wisdom.

THE NARCISSIST AT MIDLIFE

Success is a lousy teacher. It seduces smart people into thinking they can't lose.

Bill Gates

Whereas the child has to deal with individuation and the adolescent with interdependence, older adults must make peace with mortality. As we wrinkle and lose some of our energy, people with identities based on beauty and physical prowess are faced with having to discover new ways of valuing themselves. You have to jump off of your body and onto your spirit for the last act of life's journey. In other words, if we only think of ourselves as our bodies, our vitality and sense of self will decline along with our physical self. But if we can build a deeper relationship with our inner experience, the slowing down of the body can be reduced to an inconvenience.

For those whose personal identity and relationships are based on their powers of attraction, aging strikes a severe blow. A 45-year-old former fashion model once told me flatly, "You know I couldn't have survived middle age without all this therapy!" Another fragile narcissist who suffered early trauma stated, "My makeup is a core part of who I

am." For the narcissist, aging represents a series of sham-
ing experiences that can lead to deforming plastic surgeries,
immersion in fantasies of youth, or withdrawal into depressive isolation. For these people, aging is experienced as a
personal failure.

SELF-PARENTING

> *There is nothing like a dream to create the future.*
>
> Victor Hugo

Paul was in his early 50s when he came to therapy struggling
with a self-proclaimed midlife crisis. He had worked hard,
achieving success as an investment banker. Paul enjoyed the
complex puzzle presented by each new company. He had
to learn the business, identify problems, and find ways of
increasing profitability. He especially enjoyed discovering
the true financial situation of a business hidden beneath layers of creative bookkeeping. Driven by what he called perfectionism, he worked day and night, driving himself, his
partners, and employees with what he described as relentless dissatisfaction.

> Dissatisfaction, that's it! I'm dissatisfied with everything—
> myself, my colleagues, my living situation, and the women
> I meet. I'm never happy with anything I do in any area of
> my life. I was dissatisfied with being married and now I'm
> dissatisfied with being single. I'm dissatisfied with where

Parietal–Frontal Circuits

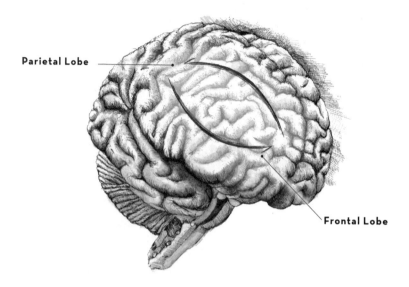

Parietal Lobe

Frontal Lobe

I've gotten in my career, and can't believe how most of the guys who I've hired, trained, and helped get established have surpassed me. They've all gone on to bigger things, are more respected, and make a lot more money. I've been passed over for promotions, been let go during downsizing, and gone from job to job trying to find the right place to use my talents. My life is half over and, so far, it feels like a bad dream that just won't stop.

Paul survived a tumultuous childhood full of pain and conflict. His mother had abused drugs, both parents were physically violent, and his father abandoned the family when

Paul was 13. It became clear to Paul that his mother was unable to care for him and his younger sister, so he took it upon himself to enroll both of them in boarding school. From as early as he could remember, he kept long hours, played and worked hard, and assumed he was destined for great things. For 25 years, his superstar identity distracted him from his emptiness and emotional pain, but turning 50 burst his bubble.

> In my mind, I'm still the young stud that was going to set the world on fire, marry a supermodel, and live in a mansion. Instead, I'm living alone in an apartment, dating women I don't respect, and struggling to pay my bills. How could I miss the reality of my life for so long? I've always lived in the fantasy of being the top dog and suddenly, it's as if I went from superstar to loser overnight. My reality sucks! Since I realized how depressed I was, I've tried to outrun it by getting up earlier, doing more deals, and working out harder, but the truth keeps catching up with me.

As a child, Paul had no guidance in how to forge an identity, get a realistic sense of his own capabilities, or learn how to cope with difficult emotions. His early narcissism, the narcissism we all share as young children, never matured into a healthy and balanced sense of self-esteem. He remained in a world of black-and-white thinking, where human value was measured against perfectionistic ideals. As a result, he was disappointed with everything and everyone, especially himself. Paul shrugged his shoulders.

> I feel like a stranger in my own life. All of a sudden I find myself at 50 with the wrong set of rules. Most of the time I'm confused about what to do and it stops me in my tracks. I still have the impulse to work hard, chase women, push myself to the limit, and try to achieve the goals that have always been before me. The difference is that I can't seem to shake the feeling that it's all meaningless.

Despite being put off by aspects of his narcissism, I felt that Paul was a remarkable man. From a hellacious early life, he not only took over the parenting of his younger sister but managed to support her and himself through graduate school. Despite his career disappointments, he knew his field well and had developed a wide range of competencies. Although his marriage had failed, he was a kind and loving person, devoted to his family and friends. His failures in both love and work appeared related to his perfectionism; he had been unable to accept anything less than an ideal world or perfect people, and he had let everyone know it. This attitude soured those around him, and he was often excluded from social get-togethers and passed over for promotions.

Paul's painful realization at 50 was learning that he was a mere mortal. He would have to come to terms with not living up to his childhood fantasies before he would be able to achieve happiness and satisfaction in his real life. Paul would

have to learn to love the real people in his life and accept the
level of performance he and those around him were capable
of attaining.

Paul's therapy experience was arduous, but he gradually
began to see through many of his illusions. In one session,
Paul asked me, "How could I have lived 50 years and missed
something so obvious, something that was right in front of
my nose the entire time?" I thought for a while before offering some thoughts. "Our inner worlds are ageless and the
defenses you developed as a young boy kept you going for
half a century. Perhaps you are finally strong enough to face
the pain of your childhood and learn to love and accept
yourself for who you are. And from what I see, you are worthy of care, respect, and love."

For many of us, later adulthood is a time when we finally
find the insight, courage, and wisdom to exorcize old demons
and learn new ways of being. As we age, we are better able
to use both hemispheres when processing information. We
come to be less driven by anxiety and we are better able to
see through the distortions, biases, and impulsivity that can
hamper us in adolescence and young adulthood. Enhancing
centeredness, self-awareness, and mindfulness lie before us
as evolutionary frontiers of consciousness.

10

Stories as Nurturance

Imagination is more important than knowledge.

—*Albert Einstein*

Have you ever sat in a café, watching people talk or chat on the phone? Ever wonder what all of the talking is about? Could everyone have that much worth saying? When sociologist Robin Dunbar eavesdropped on these conversations, he found that the vast majority of what is said is nonessential.[1] In other words, almost all our conversations have no purpose other than to keep us connected. With the evolution of culture and language, the ways we nurture one another have expanded beyond grooming, touch, and sharing food to words and stories. Although most of the content of our verbal communication is nonessential, words are a social glue and a primary connection to the group.

As social creatures, humans are constantly sharing information with one another. Given a bit more time, we share stories—our encounters with the traffic cop, a trip to the barber shop, or something we saw an adorable 3-year-old do earlier in the day. Given still more time, we may tell longer and more elaborate stories, some of which end up being told again and again. Some of these stories stick in our minds and compel us to spread them to others.

Of these stories, a few become part of group memory. These stories often embody personal struggles and moral principles that transcend time and say something important about what it means to be human. The Iliad and Bhagavad Gita come to mind as examples of stories that turn into legends and cultural cornerstones. From ancient religious texts to tweets, social information exchange never sleeps.

In order to more fully appreciate the role of storytelling in human culture, it is important to realize that the abundance of media in today's world is a recent phenomenon. Written language available to everyday people is only a few hundred years old. Throughout history, the knowledge and wisdom of a tribe were transmitted via face-to-face storytelling. For most of human evolution and in many places in the world today, oral tradition serves as the primary means of transmitting culture among individuals and across generations. Now that there are few places free of cell phone and Internet service, this will soon come to an end.

I'm in my 60s and live on the West Coast, while my mom is in her 80s and lives back East. On most weekends one of us calls the other to check in and say hi, and we spend anywhere from 10 minutes to an hour listening to each other's voices. We talk about the weather, share our various maladies, and catch up on family gossip. This week she told me about a rockslide in her town that took out a delicatessen that made good tuna sandwiches. "Too much rain—too fast—inadequate drainage," said she. I told her about my sinus problems that the doctors can't seem to diagnose. "Antibiotics don't work—no end to phlegm—inadequate drainage," said I. This apple hasn't fallen far from the tree.

At some point in the conversation, something will trigger a memory in her. "Have I ever told you about . . . " she begins, and launches into a story from the past. These stories can go on for a long time. I enjoy hearing most of them, even those I've heard before. Many of them are tales of her childhood and the travels of our many relatives. Sometimes I imagine what it must have been like to sit with one's family around the hearth in the distant past, listening to tales of tribal history.

To understand the brains of older adults who excel in telling tales from long ago, we may benefit from taking an evolutionary perspective on their abilities to better recall and recount old information rather than more recent stories. One of the many negative stereotypes of older people is that they talk too much, stray from topic to topic, and get sidetracked by irrelevant details. There is even a technical-sounding term, *off-topic verbosity*, to describe this style of communication.[2] It is generally attributed to the breakdown of cognitive filtering that keeps the elderly from inhibiting irrelevant thoughts and feelings in their communication.[3]

While there may be some truth to these pathology-based

theories, language functioning remains generally intact for the vast majority of us well into late adulthood.[4] Older adults do become less concerned with being concise as they focus on transmitting their life experiences to those around them.[5] They pay more attention to whether their audience is paying attention and will do and say things to capture a straying listener. Elders report the most satisfaction in communicating these stories when they experience the enjoyment of their listeners.[6] For older adults, storytelling is not designed to be precise or support the accomplishment of external goals, but rather is a means of transmitting history, the expansion of culture, and the pleasure of connection.

THE RACONTEUR

How pleasant is the day when we give up striving to be young—or slender.

William James

One of the best things about being a therapist is hearing lots of stories. The best are usually told by older folks who, through countless repetitions, have worked on their style and timing, and seem to enjoy telling their stories a little more each time. They set the scene, develop characters, and come in for a perfect landing on the punch line or the moral of the story. One such storyteller was Sidney, whose therapy consisted of holding court with an audience of one. Every now and then he would let me get a word in, but if I offered an alternate way of looking at something, he would dismiss me with a wave of the hand and say, "You're a kid. What do you know?" Sid would always follow this with a wink and a smile to let me know he had heard what I had said and that it was appreciated. He was a dear man.

About a year after his wife's death, Sid's son had noticed that Sid seemed distracted, disoriented, and forgetful. He feared that Sid, now 73, was suffering from the beginnings of dementia and took him to see a neurologist. These tests pointed away from dementia and toward depression, resulting in a referral for therapy, which is how Sid and I met. During our first meeting he laid down the law: "No tears, no drugs, and I'm not gonna tell you about my mother or what ink stains look like." I liked him immediately. "How about telling me about you?" I said. He took it from there.

Sidney's family had come from Eastern Europe to Chicago in the 1920s, where they started a factory machining parts for appliances and airplanes. His earliest memories were of his father bringing home small engine parts for him to play with. "He had a plan for me," Sid said, raising his index finger for emphasis. His entire family was employed at the factory and there was little separation between work and home—everything revolved around "the business." Surviving the Depression, World War II, and losing most of their family in the Holocaust only made them more diligent, thankful, and aware of the fragility of life. Needless to say, Sid never spent much time playing games or relaxing.

Other than a few years away from work, which he spent as a paratrooper in France and Italy, most of his life was spent at the factory.

"I worked hard my whole life, running a business, fighting Nazis and labor unions, trying to be tough, and I was pretty tough, let me tell you. I was always on the go, always keyed up, always worried about something. Would I make payroll? Could I pay the mortgage and the kids' tuition? Was I dressed right? Did I look good?" His eyes smiled as he said, "You wouldn't know it to look at me now, but I didn't do too bad with the ladies in my day. Someday if you're good, I'll tell you about the French girls." Another wink.

I imagine that Sid's grief over the loss of his wife had led him to withdraw from his usual activities and social connections. This evolved into a set of habits lasting long enough to alter his biology into the downward spiral of depression. Fortunately, Sid's son intervened before his depression became too deeply entrenched. I could sense that my presence, attention, and interest were part of a natural healing process that was as good as or better than the antidepressants he warned me not to suggest. It seemed that my attention had created enough leverage to help him to heal himself. As a therapist, it is good to remember that you can often help more by doing less.

By teaching me about himself and his life, Sid was reminded of how much he enjoyed interacting with other people. As our relationship deepened, I believe that he was reframing his life in the context of our attachment and a lifetime of positive memories. My curiosity helped Sid to reflect on his life and remember how interesting it was and could continue to be. I wanted to somehow encourage him to get reconnected with old friends, make new ones, visit family, take trips, and join some group activities in his community. I didn't want to prescribe these things, so I simply asked about them.

As Sid talked about his life before his wife's death, he would say things like, "I should call Sammy to see how he is," or "I bet my son would enjoy doing that again." These thoughts gradually turned into action as Sid became more energized. As he reconnected to his social network, his depressive symptoms and cognitive problems resolved. Fortunately, attachment stimulates the chemistry of positive mood and neural plasticity.

During one of our last sessions, I asked Sid what he liked best about aging. He thought long and hard before saying, "I just don't give a damn." Then he thought again for awhile before saying, "Don't get me wrong—I still care about people and I want the world to be a better place. What I don't give a damn about is all the stuff that I used to be afraid of, the stuff that kept me up at night. Not just work and money, but all the things that used to seem so important, like whether people liked me or whether I dressed right. I used to worry if I was cool! Can you imagine, *cool?* I realize now that these things mean less than nothing, and what a relief! It's a shame I wasted so much time and energy worrying about nothing. I learned in my old age that what is important is happening inside of me and within the people I love." Well said, Sid. And yes, I eventually got to hear about the French girls.

This drive toward storytelling in older adults, spurred by changes in our brains, minds, and hearts, creates models for the stories that younger people come to tell about themselves. As we age, our experience of relationships, like our stories, goes through a continual metamorphosis. For example, at age 25, 92% of the focus of our stories concern our wishes for the future and are about us. By age 60, 71% of our concerns, wishes, and hopes shift to our families, friends, and humanity.[7] The stories of the young are about shaping an identity, while those told by the old to the young are mostly meant to be a gift.

THE IMPORTANCE OF STORIES

Memory is the mother of wisdom.
Aeschylus

Contrary to our ideologies of rugged individualism, we live within a fabric of relationships that includes the stories we tell one another about ourselves and our experiences with others. The human brain coevolved with spoken language, larger, more complex social groups, and an increase in caretaking and interdependency. Within this evolutionary matrix, storytelling came to serve a variety of functions. A well-told story contains gestures, expressions, and ideas flavored with feelings, leading from conflicts to resolutions. The stories become a soundtrack that guides our behaviors and shapes our identities. Storytelling creates a sacred and timeless space in which the past and present merge in the service of the future.

Cultural memories embedded within stories and myths evolve over time. Each time a memory is accessed, it can be modified by new experiences so that it remains relevant to the present moment.[8] In fact, any caring person can modify the identity of others by helping them to edit their stories, leveraging the malleability of memory positively with each new generation.

Humans are akin to neurons communicating across a social synapse, and when loving others link up with us, the result can be a vital integration where the total is much greater than the sum of its parts. We can use our interpersonal resonance, intuition, and empathic abilities to heal one another through the telling and retelling of stories. Stories also help us remember who we are. If our self-narratives are positive and optimistic, they support well-being and mental health. If they are negative and anticipate failure, they can be damaging to our health, success, and self-image.

As human brains evolved more complex and functionally diverse neural networks, integrating these systems grew increasingly challenging. An example of this challenge is coordinating our left and right hemispheres. Originally mirror images of each other, the two sides of our brain have grown increasingly dissimilar through primate evolution. The right hemisphere specialized in the representation and organization of the body, emotional regulation, visual processing, and imagination. It also came to organize autobiographical memory and a cohesive and consistent sense of self. These functions were best served by simultaneously processing images, actions, and emotions, forming an automatic and nonverbal form of experience and the self.

On the other side of the brain, the left hemisphere came to specialize in the organization, sequencing, and planning involved in navigating the world. As social relating became more and more complex, the left hemisphere came to organize social grooming, gestures, handshakes, and eventually the development of language. It has been proposed that while the two hemispheres once held equal sway over our behavior, the left hemisphere came to organize conscious behavior and inhibit input from the right during waking hours. Although the subordination of the right hemisphere has helped us to create science and civilization, it has put us at risk of an estrangement or a lack of awareness of our emotions, intuition, and inner experience.

So what role do narratives play in the coordination and integration of brain functioning? Although heard and processed sequentially, narratives also involve gestures, expressions, emotions, and visual imagination that require the joint participation of the left and right hemispheres, cortical and subcortical networks.[9] While we usually assume that these integrative functions only occur within the brain. It is my contention that narratives support the integration of the two hemispheres and diverse neural networks. It's a way in which some of the brain's needs can be outsourced to the group mind.

I use the word *narrative* to describe the sequencing of events that drive the temporal structure of a story, its emotional background, and its underlying theme. What is the basic narrative structure of a novel, a children's book, or a Hollywood movie? It contains a central character or hero who faces a series of obstacles. Some obstacles are external, like a competition or the presence of an enemy. Other obstacles are internal, such as an inner brokenness that causes prolonged pain and thwarts the hero's ability to move forward to obtain the goal. The goal can be anything from love, to winning a game, to basic survival. In the process of the narrative, things get bad, and then get a little worse, before the challenges are ultimately faced and surpassed. As the story proceeds, heroes mature, endure suffering, and eventually find redemption.

Good stories are emotionally evocative, draw us in, and connect the audience through parallel emotions and experiences. A good story always contains conflict and trouble; of what interest is Red Riding Hood without the Big Bad Wolf, Luke Skywalker without Darth Vader, or Othello without Iago? We become part of the challenge, struggle with difficult feelings, and learn about ourselves along the way. Our attraction to these stories is not an accident; they not only provide for neural integration, but also teach us to problem solve, persevere in the face of conflict, and manage fear and uncertainty.

Our early lives are dominated by fairy tales and myths that usually contain literal and metaphoric meanings. Cinderella represents our feelings of being unappreciated; the wicked stepsisters embody the bullies in all of our lives, and Prince Charming fulfills our dreams of being loved and appreciated for who we are. The fact that many cultures have parallel stories speaks to the commonality of human experience. We process the words of the story while simultaneously experiencing the emotional ups and down with the protagonist. Because the left hemisphere is processing the semantic aspects of words while the right is processing its metaphoric meaning and emotional significance, hearing and telling stories results in simultaneous activation and integration of both hemispheres.[10]

I THINK I CAN, I THINK I CAN, I KNOW I CAN

Pessimism leads to weakness, optimism to power.

William James

A favorite story of one of my youngest clients was *The Little Engine That Could*. Joey had his parents read it as one of his bedtime rituals at every possible opportunity. Although they all knew it by heart, Joey insisted that they hold the book and turn the pages at the appropriate time. During one of our sessions, while struggling to piece together a puzzle more appropriate for older kids, I heard him quietly saying to himself, "I think I can. I think I can." Joey had internalized this story in such a way that the entire narrative—

beginning, middle, and end—could be summarized in this single brief phrase. He had learned to use it in moments of challenge to persevere through difficulties, regulate his frustration, and have confidence in a positive outcome.

Joey evoked the little train to create a state of mind that helped him face challenges. He made the story part of his internal experience that was available to him when needed. In just this way, stories become mechanisms of emotional regulation that serve to keep us calm and remain in control of our thoughts and feelings.[11] The emotional regulation they provide supports not only left-right integration but a more regulated state of arousal that supports neuroplasticity and learning, as well as a positive and optimistic mood.

The importance of narratives for brain integration may be why we find correlations between mental health, emotional regulation, and the quality of an individual's personal narratives.[12] Individuals who are able to put their stressful experiences into words and tell their stories to others experience less distress, have enhanced immunological functioning, and spend less time at the doctor's office.[13] There is evidence that narratives aid in emotional security while minimizing the need for elaborate psychological defenses.[14]

Children with more sophisticated narratives that include self-reflective remarks are more likely to be securely attached.[15] This is largely due to the fact that secure and emotionally mature parents and grandparents are aware of their own internal emotional states and share this information when talking with their children. They also ask their children what's on their minds and how they feel, offering opportunities for shared emotional learning and the coconstruction of personal narratives. Older adults not only have the time to offer this form of nurturance to children, their brains are actually primed for it.

Who do you know who likes to hear the same stories, again and again, in precisely the same way? Probably the young children in your life. And do you know anyone who likes to tell stories again and again as if they never told you before? Most likely your parents, grandparents, and other older folks in your life. The juxtaposition of these two instinctual drives is unlikely to be a coincidence. I am pretty confident that this reflects a genetically driven lock-and-key mechanism for the transmission of knowledge and wisdom across the generations from a time before written language. Storytelling, a time-honored tradition across all cultures, is something that modern technological societies should not surrender without a fight. Rather, we should find ways to foster and reinforce this ancient tradition to support biological, psychological, and spiritual health.

The widening divide between right and left hemisphere processing has increased the challenge of integrating rational thought with unconscious feelings and intuition. Stories, myths, and fables can help us cope with anxieties that cannot be dealt with by logic alone. Think of the example of hunting as a potential incubator for early myth. The rational strategies of hunting would help our ancestors successfully track and capture prey while myths and rituals would help them deal with the complex emotions involved in competition, separation from their families, and the killing of animals.

The value of stories, myths, and rituals cannot be assessed on the factual accuracy but on whether they feel true and help us to live with more courage. While logic demands consistency, accuracy, and linearity, myth uses stories as vehicles of connection to create meaning and nurture the listener. Although myths arise from the past, they represent timeless themes that continue to be a part of human experience. The myth of the hero and its eternal theme of the courage to persevere in the face of challenge is core to the survival of each individual and the tribe as a whole.

WISDOM: ATTAINED AND SUSTAINED

The growing ranks of elderly . . . will be like having a
vastly expanded senate in our civilization.

Arnold Scheibel

Just as we can now use journals, photographs, film, and other media to enhance the storage capacity of our memories, storytelling and its underlying neural structures were expanded to hold entire lives and cultures. I would be willing to wager that, over evolutionary time, narratives became a strategy for embedding information within the group mind, allowing the individual brain to grow further in size and increase in complexity.

One of my favorite examples of this came from a small coastal village rebuilding in the wake of the Indian Ocean tsunami in 2004. Although the buildings were all destroyed, rescue workers were stunned to find that all of the villagers had survived. They discovered that after the earthquake, the village matriarch told a story from her childhood about the importance of going to the mountaintop after the ground shakes. Following her advice, the tribe went to the top of the island's central mountain, watched as the tsunami washed away their village, and safely returned after the ocean receded.

As my parents grow older like their parents before them, it is impossible to escape the fact that they are storytellers. I listen, smile through each recitation, and play my designated role in the unfolding of the familiar drama. As an adolescent, I remember growing impatient hearing these stories again and again. Now the experience is a mixture of pleasure and the bittersweet awareness that I may not hear them for much longer. These stories are no longer about learning something new, but about the revitalization of memories and the enduring embrace of our common history.

Although no one was completely sure how old she was, my grandmother lived well into her 90s. Ever since I was a small child, she always had a jar of hand cream nearby, and was in an almost constant state of moisturizing. As she spoke, she would draw me closer, eventually moisturizing my hands in hers. When I visited during her last years, I would pull my chair up close to hers. She would take my hands into hers, start moisturizing, look into my eyes, and begin, "Remember the time . . . " launching into the stories of our shared past. Each visit had the same stories, smiles, smells, and touches. I think of this as a ritual space where our hearts, minds, and bodies would synchronize as we became absorbed in shared memories. We have seen that the changes that occur in the brain during the life span seem to increase bilateral processing and alter the focus of attention toward personal narrative. When wise elders tell stories, it is not only for entertainment but to provide life lessons and guidance for thought and action. Perhaps being closer to the end of life than to its beginning, older adults spin these stories in a way that urges the listener to seize the day, take risks, and appreciate life's fragile beauty.

As we progress through adolescence and into adulthood, the pressures of raising a family, establishing a career, and dealing with day-to-day realities lead us to deal with life in increasingly rational ways. As these pressures are alleviated and we gain greater perspective, we look back to recapture some of the mythic components of our past we left behind. Our children offer us the opportunity to reconnect with mythical and magical thinking and the value these tales can have for us overly rational adults.

Part
Four

BODY AND SOUL

Nurturing Your Body

*Whether we live to a vigorous old age lies
not so much in our stars or in our genes but
in ourselves.*

—George Vaillant

THE BRAIN AND BODY ARE ONE AND THE SAME. THIS
is why the health of the body is so crucial to the health of
the brain. Our closest primate ancestors were vegetarians,
spending most of the day munching on fruit and foliage. As
the brain grew, it consumed an ever-increasing percentage of
the body's energy. In fact, our brains have grown in size faster
than our bodies and use far more energy than any of our
other organs.[1]

Compared to other primates, humans have less muscle
and more fat, which we retain for our energy-hungry brains
in times of scarcity.[2] As our brain's need for energy increased,
our digestive organs actually decreased in size as we developed strategies to get more nutritiously concentrated food.[3]

The importance of nutrition necessitated a communal, multigenerational focus on hunting and gathering, and an expansion of culture around preserving and cooking food.

The deep psychic connection between emotional and caloric nurturance begins in early mother-child experiences. Human milk is low in fat, prolonging mother-infant contact and enhancing bonding and infant safety. The image of the matriarch forever standing in front of the hearth, cooking beloved specialties and family recipes transcends culture. In my travels to Africa, Europe, and the South Pacific, I'm invariably invited to join people in their homes to taste their wives', mothers', or grandmothers' cooking. The invitation is usually accompanied by a rolling of the eyes, a smacking of the lips, and a blissful expression to describe what I'm about to experience. The communal hearth is a universal symbol of nurturance and connection. Brain, body, mind, and relationships have become inextricably interwoven.

DIET

I saw few die of hunger; of eating, a hundred thousand.
                                                Benjamin Franklin

Many studies have found that restricted caloric intake has a positive effect on the brain and our ability to learn. Caloric restriction triggers a variety of brain processes supportive of healthy functioning, including decreasing the amount of

destructive oxidation within neurons. Keep in mind that
caloric restriction should not be confused with malnutri-
tion. This research was conducted in developed countries
with ready access to high-quality food, allowing participants
to obtain a balanced and vitamin-rich diet despite the low
number of calories.

I suspect that the connection between consuming fewer
calories and positive brain health may also be based in evolution. The less food we consume, the more active and alert
we need to be to find food for ourselves and our offspring.
Hunger triggers the brain and body into action; one has to
think of what to do to solve the problem of hunger—start
foraging, go hunting, and so on. With less food, there is
more exploration of the environment, covering new ter-
rain and confronting new problems to solve. This is one of
the essential tasks of survival and one of the primary functions around which the brain has evolved. As much research
shows, novelty and challenge build neural structures.

In addition to the calories we consume, the kinds of
foods we eat can also influence brain health. While diet and
the health of the body is a vast area of study, knowledge
about the specific impact of diet on the brain is limited. So
far, four links between diet and brain health have been identified (see Table 11.1). The antioxidants found in berries and
some other foods have been shown to support neural health.
Improved learning, memory, balance, strength, stamina, and
coordination all correlate with antioxidant intake.[4]

Similar positive correlations have been found from

higher levels of folic acid, which results in a better memory and greater life satisfaction, while working against symptoms of Parkinson's and Alzheimer's disease.[5] Fatty acids found in salmon and flax seeds support neural structures and reduce the risk of cognitive dysfunction and dementia.[6] And finally, soy products and legumes support memory, executive function, and hippocampal growth, and correlate with a decreased risk of Alzheimer's disease.[7]

Table 11.1. The Effects of Diet on the Brain

Chemical Compound	Impact on Neural Structures	Found In
Antioxidants[a]	Increased hippocampal plasticity Enhanced dopamine functioning Reduction of neuronal lesions and inflammation	Blueberries, strawberries, spinach, grapes
Folic acid[b]	Enhanced neuronal self-repair Increased neural longevity	Whole wheat, leafy greens, liver, oranges, and asparagus
Essential fatty acids[c]	Maintenance and health of cell membranes Proper central nervous system functioning	Salmon, flaxseed, soybean oil, and walnuts
Phytoestrogen[d]	Increased vascular health and functioning Hippocampal neurogenesis	Broccoli, berries, and soy products

EXERCISE

After 30, your body has a mind of its own.

Bette Midler

The idea of a connection between a healthy mind and a healthy body goes back at least to the Greek gymnasium, where they were thought of as one and the same. It was later, under the influence of Christianity, that the separation of mind and body became woven into our philosophy.

When the body is active, it signals the brain to be on alert and ready to learn and grow. As such, the brain needs to be on alert to maximize the probability of success. Neural networks dedicated to action, perception, and cognition evolved together over millions of years and develop together during our lifetimes. Because of their interdependence, physical activity exerts a stimulating influence on the brain that keeps it functioning at an optimal level. Our movement through space signals the brain to predict and control environmental contingencies, keep us safe from predators, and be on the alert for food and potential mates. Thus, intelligence is a full-body proposition, and physical activity stimulates our intellects.

Aerobic exercise pumps more oxygen through the brain and enhances the health of the capillaries through which it flows.[8] This is why active adults have better blood supply to their brains and experience fewer of the small strokes so common later in life. Exercise also triggers a cascade of biological processes that support brain health, plasticity, and learning. Athletes have been found to possess higher levels of glial cells, endorphins, dopamine, serotonin, and nor-epinephrine that elevate mood, self-esteem, and cognitive processing. In addition, exercise stimulates a wide range of genetic transcriptional processes that support brain health, longevity, and immunological functioning.[9]

These benefits include better attentional capacities, exec-utive control, visuospatial abilities, and slower memory loss. Benefits also include decreased incidence of cognitive decline, dementia, and psychiatric symptoms. Exercise and caloric restriction both appear to trigger enhanced attention, energy, and learning. They give the brain the message that we need food, and that action and new learning are required to survive—exactly the message we want to send to our brains. The brain receives the opposite message when we rely on Ubers to take us from restaurant to restaurant for calorie-rich meals.

SLEEP

It's useless to play lullabies for those who can't sleep.

John Cage

If you have ever experienced sleep deprivation, then you have no doubt that sleep is "by the brain and for the brain" and is absolutely required for healthy neural functioning.[10] Research has found that sleep deprivation results in deficits in memory, attention, concentration, problem solving and mood.

Approximately 5% of the transcription genes in the cerebral cortex change their level of expression between waking and sleeping states. Those activated during wakefulness are involved in energy metabolism, excitatory neurotransmission, synaptic activation, memory acquisition, and neural response to stress. Gene transcription related to sleep includes those involved in protein synthesis, synaptic consolidation, and myelin formation.[11] These findings show us that the different genes activated during waking and sleeping are complementary and essential for memory organization and the maintenance of neural health.

Scientists have long suspected that neural connections are remodeled during sleep in order to consolidate memory—a process by which new memories are moved to long-term storage.[12] In almost all studies involving learning and memory, performance improves after a nap or a good night's sleep and decreases precipitously with sleep deprivation.[13] Sleep deprivation has been shown to have a persisting negative effect on hippocampus-dependent conscious memory and that longer periods of rapid eye movement (REM) sleep enhanced emotional memory formation.[14]

Sleep may also support insight and new ideas, as it did for at least two prominent scientists. The neuroscientist Otto Loewi recalled waking up in the middle of the night having come upon the idea that neurons communicate via chemical neurotransmitters. In a similar fashion, Dmitri Mendeleev conceived of the idea of organizing the elements according to atomic weights in a dream and, when

he awoke, created the periodic table.[15] In one study, subjects were presented with a cognitive task on which they
could improve gradually by increasing response speed or
dramatically by gaining insight into the abstract rules. Initial training was followed by 8 hours of either wakefulness
or sleep. During the next session, more than twice as many
subjects gained insight after sleep than after equal periods
of wakefulness.[16]

Although it is commonly believed that we need less sleep
as we grow older, we actually need as much sleep as ever.
What diminishes is not our need for sleep, but our ability
to fall asleep and stay asleep through the night.[17] Because
sleep deprivation has been shown to have moderate to severe
effects on attention, concentration, and memory at any age,
sleep disorders should always be explored first when adults
are experiencing cognitive difficulties.[18] This is especially
true for older adults, given that more than half of people
over 65 experience some form of a sleep problem.[19]

The majority of sleep disturbances in older adults, such
as broken sleep and apnea, are secondary to other changes
that go along with normal aging. Sleep disturbances are also
associated with heart and lung disease, arthritis, stroke,
anxiety, and depression, as well as the medications used
to treat them. Retirement, decreased physical activity, and
lack of a regular schedule can also contribute to sleep problems. Psychosocial factors such as isolation, loneliness, and
bereavement are also known to promote sleep disturbances
in older adults.[20]

Sleep apnea, or breathing-related sleep disturbance, has reported prevalence rates as high as 45–62% for people over 60.[21] Those who suffer with apnea will have anywhere from dozens to hundreds of breathing lapses and sleep interruptions throughout the night. Although people are often unaware that they suffer from apnea, they experience frequent brief awakenings during the night and feel tired in the morning.[22]

Biochemical changes associated with normal brain aging increase our vulnerability to sleep disturbances. With age, we also experience decreasing levels of melatonin and prolactin, which regulate circadian rhythm, as well as neural loss in brain structures that controls our sleep-wake cycle.[23] These changes result in an advanced sleep-wake cycle that makes us sleepy in the early evening hours and wakes us up in the early morning. This pattern of sleep leads to less restorative and dream (REM) sleep, more awakenings during the night, and less total time asleep.

BETTER SLEEP

Dreams pass into the reality of action. From the actions stem the dream again; and the interdependence produces the highest form of living.

Anaïs Nin

It is clear that getting a good night's rest is a critical component of maintaining a healthy brain. Following some basic guidelines for improving sleep is a good idea at any age. Some rules for better sleep throughout adulthood include limiting naps, taking a daily walk, watching the effect of medications on sleep, avoiding caffeine, especially after lunch, and limiting liquids in the evening. See Table 11.2 for a more complete set of suggestions.

Table 11.2. Rules for Better Sleep [a]

Limit naps to 30 minutes in the early afternoon	Exercise daily
Increase exposure to sunlight later in the day	Limit liquids in the evening
Check the effect of medications on sleep	Avoid heavy meals in the evening
Avoid caffeine, alcohol, and tobacco after lunch	Eat a light snack before bed
Go to bed and arise at the same time every day	Get out of bed if not able to sleep
Create a quiet, dark, comfortable place to sleep	Develop a relaxing bedtime ritual
Avoid thinking about life issues while trying to fall asleep	

In addition to good sleep hygiene, a number of other options are available. Melatonin, a naturally occurring chemical in our bodies that regulates our sleep-wake cycle, decreases with age. Available at health food and grocery stores, melatonin supplements have been shown to help many people fall asleep, stay asleep longer, and decrease the number of awakenings during the night. Bright light therapy used late in the day has effects similar to taking melatonin.[24]

Machines that assist in maintaining continuous airway pressure (CPAP and BIPAP), as well as behavioral and pharmacological interventions, have also proven effective.[25] Overall, we need to keep our bodies healthy if we want optimal performance and longevity from our brains. Paying attention to diet, exercise, and sleep appears to be essential for achieving this goal, not just for the older old, but for all of us.

ONE HUNDRED PLUS

None are so old as those who have outlived enthusiasm.

Henry David Thoreau

Just a few decades ago, it was relatively rare to celebrate someone's 100th birthday, but this is changing fast. The 50,000 centenarians counted in the 1995 U.S. Census was a 3,000% increase over the 1952 census. The number of centenarians worldwide in 1998, 135,000, is predicted to grow to 2.2 million by 2050.[26] These exceptionally old individuals live up to 25 years beyond the average life span. Their ability to delay or escape age-related diseases, such as dementia, stroke, cancer, cardiovascular disease, and diabetes, is of great interest to researchers. Their resistance to illness suggests a particularly successful set of genetic, immunological, and emotional defenses against many normal processes of aging.[27]

Of course, successful extreme aging involves more than the avoidance of terminal illnesses; it also requires the maintenance of cognitive and physical functioning and sustained engagement in relationships and productive activities.[28] In these domains, centenarians from around the world surprise us with high levels of energy, enthusiasm, and independence.[29] People who reach their 100th birthdays tend to live independently and in good health through their 90s, with a rapid decline near the end of life.[30]

Most researchers note that centenarians are extraordinary individuals, possessing optimism as well as "special and vibrant" qualities.[31] They also seem to be less neurotic and more conscientious, which is likely tied to a combination of lower levels of stress and a healthy lifestyle.[32] Another finding is that centenarians are more extroverted and have higher morale, indicative of reaching out to others, giving and receiving support, and maintaining attachments.[33] Italian centenarians report greater satisfaction with their families, social relationships, and life in general.[34] So is there a centenarian personality? As the number of people reaching their 100th birthday expands, future research may discover additional centenarian secrets from which we may all benefit.

12

Nurturing Relationships

Human beings are not meant to be
solitary animals.
    —J. W. Rowe and R. L. Kahn

THE MOVEMENT OF OUR BODIES AND THE ACTIVA-
tion of our senses keep our brains active and growing. In
fact, if we are deprived of physical activity and external
input, we soon become disoriented and disorganized to the
point of psychosis. For the brain to function normally, it
depends upon constant interaction with and stimulation
from the environment.

Given that our mental abilities depend on intact senses,
cognitive declines can result from a loss of hearing, vision,
or motor abilities. Studies of older adults have found that
declines in the speed and accuracy of sensorimotor functioning accounted for the majority of changes in intellectual abilities.[1] And when speed is controlled for during intelligence

testing, many of the differences between younger and older individuals disappear.[2]

Older adults often report having a harder time hearing what is said and tracking the topic being discussed. All of these experiences could be accounted for by diminished vision and hearing that taxes our mental processes and makes communication less automatic. Support for this idea comes from the fact that older adults benefit more from multisensory input, which compensates for a loss in any particular sensory input. Watching others speak and being able to see them clearly adds information from facial expressions and body gestures that reinforce spoken messages.[3] For many, language functioning may remain intact and even improve with age, but failing senses can make them more difficult to use.

Gradually deteriorating vision and hearing often go unnoticed by both individuals and those around them. On the other hand, disorientation and memory loss often result in trips to the neurologist, with everyone assuming that their sensory systems are functioning normally.[4] Patterns of falling in older adults, often a focus of medical concern, may also be the result of unrecognized declines in sensory, motor, or vestibular functioning.[5] Because decreased sensory stimulation results in decreased brain activity, it is extremely important that failing senses in older adults be diagnosed and remedied as quickly as possible. By attending to and maximizing the functioning of our bodies and sense organs, we can protect and enhance our brains' health and longevity. And of all the experiences we need to survive and thrive, it is the experience of relating to others that is the most meaningful and important.

SEE ME, FEEL ME, TOUCH ME, HEAL ME

Nothing we use or hear or touch can be expressed in words that equal what is given by the senses.

Hannah Arendt

For infants, the eyes of their parents are points of reflexive orientation and play a significant role in initial bonding. During early infancy, exciting interactions that include direct eye gaze stimulate the brain to grow. Escalating positive interactions activate dopaminergic and opioid systems, the reflection of which can be witnessed in the delight children and adults take in games of peekaboo. Thanks to the neurochemistry of bonding, the smiles and laughter elicited from a child during peekaboo and other games are addicting for both parent and child. Each time the wide eyes and smiling face reappear, there is a surge of brain activity and good feelings all around.

While somewhat speculative, it is very likely that these same reciprocal and stimulating interactions optimize brain activity and health throughout life. Face-to-face engagements with others send important messages across the social synapse that stimulate our brains to grow and learn. Visual connection usually includes storytelling which serves to organize our memories. Instead of the passive witnessing of television or watching people from a distance, face-to-face contact calls upon the structures of our social brains to engage in the dance of communication and connects to the group mind. Social engagement tells our brains that we are still part of the tribe and still needed and cared about by others. This is likely why the neural networks involved in face recognition, emotional expression, and empathy are sustained throughout life.

There is no doubt that we are social animals that need contact for both physical and emotional stimulation. In both captivity and the wild, primates spend considerable time grooming one another. While on the surface it looks as if they are protecting one another from the potentially harmful effects of insects, this is only half the story. Grooming also provides physical proximity and touch, which may be more to the point of why it is such a popular pastime. While we no longer rely on grooming for contact, all of us still require touch. Ask a widow what it is like to sleep alone after a lifetime of sharing a bed.

For most of us, being touched feels wonderful. Scratching, tickling, caressing, cuddling, and sexual touch are all central to human communication. Children hang onto their parents, lovers become entangled, and after decades of marriage it still feels good to hold hands. When others are in pain, we instinctively move toward them with physical expressions of warmth and comfort, offering a hug or simply placing a hand on their shoulder. Soothing touch calms us and decreases stress.

Our skin, the body's largest sense organ, contains two types of sensory receptors. One type transmits information that helps us locate, identify, and manipulate objects, while the second activates social and emotional brain networks.[6] This system stimulate attachment, hormonal activation, and sexual responses to affectionate and comforting caresses. While I love having my back scratched, it just doesn't feel as good when I do it myself. Besides the fact that some spots are impossible to reach, touch actually feels better when someone else touches us.[7]

The soft touch and comfortable warmth of being held triggers the secretion of oxytocin and endorphins, which lead to mild sedation and decreases in blood pressure. These biochemical processes enhance social bonding through the association of another's touch with feelings of well-being.[8] Physical contact seems especially important for preterm infants, who cry less, gain more weight, sleep better, and are discharged earlier from the hospital if they are held and massaged.[9] These mechanisms support connection and group cohesion by reinforcing us for seeking proximity and contact with other members of our tribe.

Touch is an important source of social sensory stimulation and a vital mechanism of early brain building. Increased touch results in more exploratory behavior in infancy and childhood, increased attachment security, better memory, and better parenting skills when full grown.[10] Touch also results in lower levels of stress hormones in the bloodstream and enhanced neuronal survival.[11] Patients with cancer and

other illnesses who receive therapeutic massage benefit
via the increased levels of dopamine, serotonin, oxytocin,
endorphins, and natural killer cells.[12] Both aggressive adolescents and agitated elderly show less negative symptoms
when they receive regular massage.[13] Touching can be an
increasingly important means of comfort and connection,
especially for older adults whose other sensory modalities
may be decreasing.[14]

Depressed mothers tend to touch and interact with their
children less, and, in turn, their children become more difficult
to soothe.[15] Studies have found that teaching depressed mothers to massage their infants increased the amount of touching
and bonding time between them and decreased levels of stress
hormones in both infants and mothers. These infants showed
increased alertness, emotionality, and sociability and were
easier to soothe.[16] Touching their children not only activated
smiles and positive expressions on the part of the infants, but
also made the mothers feel happier and more effective.[17]

Younger people often avoid touching older people out
of social distance, prejudice, or even physical repulsion.
And as people grow older, they may also tend to touch each
other less—an unfortunate consequence of losing those
closest to them. The power of touch is also active when we
pet our pets. In fact, the same centers in our brains—and
our cats' and dogs'—are stimulated during physical contact.[18] Pets have been shown to help us recover from organ
transplantation, during cancer treatment, in coping with
bereavement, and in the general reduction of stress.[19] People

with pets tend to move around more, suffer less depression, and have higher survival rates after heart attacks.[20] So find a pet who likes to cuddle. How can we enhance our opportunities to benefit from touching and being touched? Be strategic—volunteer in hospitals to hold preterm infants or help new mothers struggling with postpartum depression. Get massages and trade back rubs with others. Go out dancing, take martial arts classes, and engage in activities that involve movement and touch. There are all kinds of ways to increase your physical contact. Do it—it's good for you and those you touch.

WHEN YOU'RE SMILING

Wrinkles should merely indicate where smiles have been.

Mark Twain

Like touch, laughter is good medicine. Laughter stimulates our brains by increasing heart rate, blood pressure, and muscle activity.[21] This is why prolonged and hearty laughter can actually tire us out. Laughter helps us cope with stress by both decreasing cortisol levels and stimulating the production of important components of our immunological systems such as T cells, natural killer cells, and B cells.[22] Laughter and the biological processes it stimulates have even been shown to alter the expression of 23 separate genes, reflecting its power to influence the brain and body.[23]

One reason why humor and laughter feel so good is that they stimulate dopamine production, which serves to reduce anxiety, depression, and loneliness while increasing energy, hope, self-esteem, and a sense of empowerment.[24] Laughter and humor are good when we are alone but best when shared with others. Laughter is a social phenomenon and is even contagious, demonstrated by the fact that we tend to laugh more when watching a comedy with a group than when we are alone.

Freud considered humor to be one of the most mature of all of the defense mechanisms. Like other defenses, it helps us to cope with psychic pain by allowing for emotional distance and perspective on uncontrollable circumstances.[25] In addition to its defensive functions, it also has many other psychological benefits such as increased hope and optimism. Humor can play an active role in the healing process for patients with life-threatening diseases by enhancing mood, improving pain thresholds, and lessening anxiety and discomfort.[26] Older adults who use humor on a regular basis demonstrate less emotional and psychological stress.

Humor has been identified as useful in creating a feeling of connection in nursing homes and hospices for residents and staff.[27] Not only is humor present in the majority of nurse-patient interactions, but it is more likely to be initiated by the patient than the nurse.[28] Another study found a positive correlation between humor appreciation and longevity.[29] Humor may correlate with a sense of autonomy and self-efficacy by increasing our perception of control over our environment. If we can't control certain events in our lives, finding humor in our situation enhances a sense of perspective and control of life's chaos.

THE TIES THAT BIND US

From caring comes courage.

Lao Tzu

The need to belong to a group and attach to others is a fundamental human motivation.[30] Animals that evolved in groups, such as ourselves, can only be fully understood in the context of their relationships. Pack animals are linked to one another via social brain networks and use each other to regulate their internal biochemistry as well as their emotions, thoughts, and behaviors. The importance of these connections is often clearest when they are ruptured. For example, if the matriarch of a herd of elephants is killed by human hunters (which is often the case), the testosterone levels of the herd's adolescent males skyrocket, making them more aggressive and dangerous to humans.[31] Perhaps in a similar manner, fractured families and environmental stress seem to correspond to a greater level of adolescent aggression and the formation of gangs.

Because we are interconnected social organs, our relationships serve to regulate our physical health and emotional well-being. Secure attachment to supportive, kind, and caring others makes us happier, healthier, and longer lived.[32] This is why the positive correlations between health and social connectedness are the most consistent and robust findings in psychoneuroimmunology, the study of relationships between the mind, brain, and bodily health.[33] Positive social support is associated with better mental health, cardiovascular health, immunological functioning, and cognitive performance.

Social support not only has healthy effects in itself but also buffers us against future stress.[34] Supportive attachments, whether between parents and children, husbands and wives, or just between friends, provides security and reduces anxiety.[35] Being around supportive family members and friends has been shown to reduce blood pressure, autonomic and cardiovascular reactivity, and decreases the risk of illness.[36] Social support also decreases the production of stress hormones, while facilitating the production of protein-based structures such as T cells and natural killer cells that promote immune functioning.

For social support to promote health, it has to provide a sense of belonging and allow older adults to continue to feel competent, important, and efficacious.[37] Social support enhances well-being if it makes us feel cared for, esteemed by others, and a member of a network of mutual obligations.[38] Positive relationships may serve as a buffer against both chronic and acute stress, thereby enhancing both health and longevity.[39] Social support appears to slow many processes related to brain and body aging.[40] See Table 12.1 for an overview of the benefits of social support.

Table 12.1. Benefits Associated With Positive Social Support

Cardiovascular Health

General heart health[a]

Lower blood pressure[b]

Lower levels of serum cholesterol[c]

Lower cardiovascular reactivity to stress[d]

Decreased risk of fatal coronary heart disease[e]

Higher post-heart attack survival rates[f]

Immunological Functioning

Higher level of natural killer cells[g]

Improved immunological functioning[h]

Lower urinary cortisol[i]

General Health Status

Increased health status and well-being[j]

Decrease in symptom display[k]

Decreased vulnerability to clinical illness[l]

Decreased risk of cancer recurrence[m]

Mental Health

Better all-around mental health[n]

Decreased depression in the elderly[o]

Better emotional regulation[p]

Decreased depression and anxiety[q]

Less bereavement depression in men[r]

Cognitive Functioning and Related Functions

Less severe cognitive decline with age[s]   Better sleep[t]

Married people tend to live longer than single people, as do people who are members of social organizations and those who have intimate friends and broader social support networks. In a study of over 7,000 subjects, it was found that people with more social ties live longer regardless of their socioeconomic status, smoking, drinking, exercise, or obesity.[41] These findings support the fact that relationships serve our physical health by regulating our emotions, metabolism, and immunological functioning.

In decades past, it was found that married men were more financially successful in their careers than those who were unmarried. This phenomenon, known as the *marriage premium*, is reflected in an estimated 15–27% gain in income for married men over those who stay single, and a 12% gain in income for divorced men who remarry over those who remain divorced.[42] For divorced men who stay divorced, the marriage premium is lost.[43] The marriage premium has even been found in cases of shotgun weddings (forced marriage due to conception) and has also been found to exist with unmarried but cohabitating couples.[44]

Recently widowed men experience greater anxiety, and people over 65 with no social ties are more likely to experience cognitive decline.[45] Considerable evidence suggests that the risk of death is greater for people with less social contact and support and those grieving the loss of a loved one.[46] This is certainly consistent with all that we have seen about the power of sensory and interpersonal stimulation.

Sometimes people can be lonelier in bad relationships than they are in isolation. Troubled marriages result in higher levels of stress hormones and suppressed immunological functioning than social isolation, especially in women.[47] Although broad social support and close relationships are just about always good for us, critical and hostile others are bad for our health.[48] The presence of negative relationships has been found to correlate with exacerbations and relapses of psychiatric illnesses, while marital conflict and hostility have been found to have an adverse impact on different aspects of brain chemistry.[49]

Unhealthy environments, such as those that are chronically stressful, conflictual, and abusive, create unhealthy brains and bodies.[50] And when individuals are stressed by the combination of caring for others and not receiving significant support themselves, their immunological health can be significantly compromised.[51] The maintenance of abrasive, critical, and hostile close relationships takes its toll on immunological functioning, health, and longevity.[52] Hostile interactions between married people have been found to impair immunological functioning, increase stress hormone levels, and actually slow the healing of wounds.[53] In fact, some believe that the destructive effects of negative relationships may be stronger than the benefits of positive relationships.[54]

A leading theory of the 20th century described a gradual disengagement from others as a natural part of aging. Nothing in my experience as a therapist supports this theory. It is true that older adults have a greater likelihood of experiencing loneliness than their younger counterparts. Factors such as an empty nest, retirement, bereavement, and physical limitations can all result in isolation and may be more difficult to overcome with increasing age. But in every instance where I have encountered social withdrawal in older clients, it has been an expression of physical limitations, psychological distress, or both, not a loss of desire to connect with others. While a regular dose of solitude can make an important contribution to emotional balance and self-awareness, imposed isolation can be painful, debilitating, and worse. Isolation, loneliness, and depression have been shown to have a synergistic effect in diminishing well-being that results in reduced autonomic regulation, cardiac health, and immunological functioning.[55]

MAY HE REST IN PEACE

The secret of a happy marriage remains a secret.

Henny Youngman

Men currently have shorter life spans than women and are often older than the women they marry. These two facts lead many women to be condemned to long periods of widowhood. Or are they? About 10 years ago, I had an eye-opening experience at a cozy Parisian restaurant, famous for its great soufflés. A friend and I were enjoying drinks while anticipating the arrival of our meals when, with a flurry of commotion, a group of six expressive Italian women were installed at the next table. In the French style, we ignored their arrival as best we could and continued our conversation. Although we tried to keep our conversation going, my dinner partner kept smiling and breaking into laughter in response to what she was overhearing from the next table. Eventually she leaned forward to quietly fill me in on their conversation.

Apparently, the women were lifelong friends from Milan, visiting Paris as part of a celebration—the death of the last remaining husband. My friend and I tried to continue our private conversation but, too intrigued to stop eavesdropping, she finally began an ongoing translation. Soon both of us were laughing along with the group and began to smile and nod in their direction. The group quickly included us in their conversation, and we eventually joined their dinner party.

Over the course of the evening, I learned that these six gals had grown up and gone to school together, been in each others' wedding parties, and helped to raise each others' children. Over the years, one by one, their husbands had died off—accidents, illnesses, and old age—one had even been killed by his mistress. Two months before our dinner, the sixth husband had eaten his last cannoli. As part of his last words to his soon-to-be widow, he gave her permission to remarry. "Are you kidding?" she shouted to the group. "There will never be another man for me!" The double meaning of this phrase brought a roar of laughter from our table and dirty looks from those sitting around us. What made me laugh the hardest was that whenever one of them would mention the name of one of their husbands, they would all lift their glasses and together say, "May he rest in peace." It seemed clear that the last thing any of these women wanted was another husband. They had paid their dues, done their duty, and earned their freedom.

The general flavor of the conversation portrayed men as immature; needing their egos stroked and help picking out their clothes. They were worthless around the house, had little patience with the children, and needed help to find things right in front of them. Alas, men were no prize, rather burdens to be tolerated for the sake of the family. These women had come to the city of romance to celebrate their liberation from marriage.

For years, the band of six had been planning African safaris, shopping on Rodeo Drive, and walking the Great Wall of China. A few had homes in different countries, which would now become additional destination points for the group. Listening to them made me remember how I felt when I first went to college—the friends, the adventure, so many things to look forward to. Who ever thinks of a group of older women going out to explore the world?

Despite the gaiety and a considerable quantity of wine, there was a bittersweet flavor to the evening. I'm sure that these women cared for and missed their husbands and that some part of their bravado was a way to cope with loss. At the same time, there was a great deal of genuine love and enthusiasm about their relationships and future together. To say I felt like the odd man out was both figuratively and literally true—a bit like having a preview of my own funeral. It didn't help that they expressed mock pity for my unfortunate choice of gender and lack of linguistic abilities. At the same time, my evening with the Milanese six reinforced my belief that there are many ways to grow old.

Listening to their conversation made me think about how much of what they said about men is actually true. They didn't talk about their husbands as if they were wise men, but rather self-centered children in adult bodies. However, I also wondered how much these women's limited expectations of their husbands shaped the men their husbands had become. Did they allow their husbands to be involved in child care, deal with emotions, and struggle with intimacy, or did both partners simply fall into stereotypical roles?

Is it possible that the women colluded with their husbands' immaturity to make themselves feel superior and more in control of the family? How many families have I worked with in which no one confronted the father with their feelings or told him about anything unsettling because everyone assumed the truth would kill him? Women are generally better at dealing with emotions and tolerating pain, but is this difference made worse by cultural norms and gender roles? Part of building and maintaining a successful support system for physical and mental health is pushing those around you to rise to the challenge of supporting you. Asking for help and experimenting with new, expanded, and more flexible roles can be empowering. Give it a try—the results may surprise you.

13

Compassion in Action

I am what survives me.

—Erik Erikson

IN HIS SONG "GRANDMA'S HANDS," BILL WITHERS
shared memories of his grandmother clapping her hands in
church, picking him up when he fell, and saving him from a
spanking. A series of "touching" images leave no doubt of
the strength of their attachment. At the end, Bill pledges,
"When I get to heaven, I'll look for Grandma's hands."
Grandparenting is grounded in this kind of deep emotional
bond that he so beautifully describes in a series of instances
of love, care, and protection.

When the French historian and sociologist Alexis de
Tocqueville traveled across America in 1831, he described
what he saw as an ethic of the grandparents' role (and
right) to spoil their grandchildren. This often occurred, he
noted, to the surprise and dismay of the parents caught in
the middle. Some theorists think that what de Tocqueville

witnessed has a sociopolitical basis. Indulgent grandparents are often found in cultures where power is passed on from grandparent to parent while grandparents are still alive. The close relationships between grandchildren and their grandparents are thought to be fostered by grandparents' need to maintain some form of authority.[1]

This view suggests that the strong emotional bond between grandparent and grandchild serves as a means of ensuring the social position of the grandparents and limiting the power of parents over their children. As I mentioned earlier, grandparents and grandchildren may get along so well because they share a common enemy. A more appealing explanation is that once grandparents pass power to their children, they are able to be less authoritarian, more emotionally available, and more nurturing of their grandchildren. This may represent a social and emotional parallel to the grandmother gene, believed to support the health and survival of grandchildren, as discussed previously.

THE VALUE OF GRANDPARENTING

Friends are for when your grandchildren aren't available.

Anonymous

Many grandparents say that they enjoy being with their grandchildren more than they enjoyed parenting their own kids. Some say it's wonderful that they can play with them all day and get a full night's sleep after they leave. Others

say that having a broader perspective and getting less emotionally activated than they did with their own children
allows for more pleasurable relationships. Grandparents
also describe how less outside pressure allows them to relax
and enjoy their grandchildren.

In most cases, there is less discipline and more positive
affection. While children are busy rebelling against their
parents, grandparents and grandchildren can establish a
conspiratorial alliance to help navigate challenging family
dynamics and personalities. If handled in a balanced and
mature way, this can help a child to experience and express
greater emotional depth as well as learn valuable negotiation
skills. In-depth studies of the value of grandparenting for
grandchildren reveal a number of important factors across
psychological, social, and cultural domains. Grandparents
can offer a secure, constant, and loving relationship second
only to parents and provide an anchor of family connections. The presence of grandparents also provides a role
model for adulthood and aging as well as a sense of cultural
and historical rootedness.[2]

Grandparents' ability to provide these functions
depends upon their sense of commitment to the family, as
well as the extent to which they share space, time, and activities with their grandchildren. Unfortunately, older adults
are sometimes given the message that they are no longer an
integral part of their families. They are told in many ways
not to be a burden to their children and grandchildren or
interfere in their lives. The argument to get out of the way

often overshadows the more traditional continued contribution to the family.

Given the increasing longevity of older adults, grandparents are able to contribute more and more to their families. This growing ability to provide nurturance comes at a time in history when it is sorely needed. The single-family household is now the most prevalent context of child rearing in the United States. In America, 40% of babies are now being born to single mothers, while two-parent families are under increasing financial pressure to have two incomes.[3] A growing cost of modern society is the increasing absence of the father, and more recently the mother, from the moment-to-moment experience of children. Three-generation households, while common in agricultural and third-world societies, account for only 3% of contemporary American families.[4] Day care, after-school programs, and nannies now fill the nurturance gap created by nuclear families with two working parents.

Traditional cultures around the world have always included elders of both genders in a variety of social and practical tasks that are fully integrated into the life of the tribe. In addition to cooking and child care, older women take part in storytelling, ritual healing, and spiritual leadership. In some tribes, older men participate in child care in addition to their responsibilities for religious leadership, the performance of rituals, and communicating with deceased elders. These functions are not trivial; they are necessary for the physical, emotional, and spiritual survival of the tribe.

In the Tallensi tribe of West Africa, being a grandparent is considered a person's highest achievement and a prerequisite for elder status.[5]

Study after study has shown that grandparents both provide and receive a great deal of benefit by retaining their role as fully contributing members of the family. They offer emotional nurturance to their grandchildren while continuing to be active parents to their own children. There is little doubt that grandparents and other older adults are in a position to contribute to their families by filling the ever-widening gap between children's needs and parental availability.[6] Although the need for their participation is increasing, elders are being guided by cultural expectations to become increasingly distant from their families.

FILLING THE NURTURANCE GAP

A grandchild is a miracle, but a renewed relationship with your own children is an even greater one.

T. Berry Brazelton

When your children begin having children, they (and your future grandchildren) need you as much as ever. New mothers need to be supported and scaffolded by those around them as they nurture their children.[7] Minimizing their stress and nurturing a calm and receptive state of mind contributes to the growth and well-being of the next generation. Young children especially need the physical and emotional scaffolding of their mothers to optimize the brain-building process. Giving adult children breaks from child care and providing grandchildren with stimulating and loving interactions adds to the well-being the entire family.

Keep in mind that maternal stress during pregnancy negatively affects the developing brain by altering neurotransmitter levels, disturbing cerebral lateralization, and decreasing brain growth.[8] Anxious women tend to have newborns with lower levels of serotonin, dopamine, and vagal tone, all of which correlate with depression, anxiety, and attachment difficulties.[9]

A mother with postpartum depression lacks the energy to interact with and stimulate her children at the time when they most need attuned engagement.[10] Depression that manifests as irritability and anger will certainly interfere with a mother's ability to attune to her child.[11] Children of depressed mothers have also been found to experience a disruption in the development, connection, and integration of the frontal lobes. For these children, neural activation becomes biased toward the right hemisphere and puts them at increased risk for poor self-control, lower academic performance, and less empathic abilities.[12]

The prevalence and impact of postpartum depression make it a significant public health issue that grandparents are in a good position to recognize.[13] Pregnant women who receive more social support experience easier labors and less postpartum depression. Further, their babies have higher birth weights and are more developed at birth.[14] Therefore, your presence supports both your daughter's well-being and the healthy development of your grandchild's brain. On the one hand, grandparents can assist their children in getting the professional help they require to address debilitating psychiatric symptoms. On the other, they can continue to provide their grandchildren with the love and attention required for healthy brain development during sensitive developmental periods.

MEN AS NURTURERS

> Old age is the most unexpected thing that can happen
> to a man.
>
> Trotsky

While a mother's role as a nurturer is seldom questioned, and a grandmother is usually considered a competent and capable backup, the nurturing capabilities of fathers and grandfathers are often suspect. At worst, fathers do little more than pay the bills, and grandfathers are the old guys who doze off on the sofa. This perception of men in American society is captured in popular television shows of family life. While single young men are sexy and interesting, and possess unlimited potential, married men are presented as caricatures of masculinity gone wrong. From Ralph Cramden to Homer Simpson, middle-aged and older men are often portrayed as selfish adolescents. Many families accept this perspective and see their fathers and grandfathers as incompetent caretakers, but there is another reality of male nurturance beneath this prejudice.[15]

Men are not passive observers of parenthood; in fact, fathers also experience hormonal changes in response to becoming parents. Both expectant mothers and fathers show higher levels of prolactin and cortisol just before birth, while fathers show lower levels of testosterone, estradiol, and cortisol after their babies are born.[16] These data suggest that both parents are biologically attuned to the arrival of their child. In studies where available time is controlled for, the involvement of fathers is equal to that of mothers, while in single-parent homes of both genders, there is no difference in the affection reported by parents and children for one another.[17] Although this research has not been done with grandfathers, I suspect the same fundamental human processes are occurring.

So what do men contribute to their children? The answers are likely to be complex and controversial. Most research finds that men and women relate differently to children. Men are generally seen as more challenging and physically active, filling roles complementary to the calmer emotional base provided by mothers and grandmothers.[18] This style of parenting often leads fathers to be less involved with their daughters as they grow up because they aren't sure what they have to offer them. This may be why girls who have brothers receive more attention from their fathers.[19]

The value of the father's contribution to his children's

development is unmistakable. Studies have shown that a dad's involvement in caretaking is predictive of secure attachment.[20] The quality of father-child attachment predicts things like social competence, social adjustment, self-esteem, and school adjustment.[21] Among school-aged children, positive male engagement results in greater self-control, life skills, and social competence, which persisted through adolescence.[22] As playmates, fathers and grandfathers stimulate cognitive and social growth, and their positive availability to children is associated with better social skills, academic performance, emotional regulation, and moral development.[23]

There is not a great deal of research specifically focused on the importance of grandfathers to the development and well-being of their adult children and grandchildren. There is, however, considerable research into the impact of fathers and stepfathers that we can use to understand the importance of grandfathers. Fathers and stepfathers have been found to have an equally positive effect on their children's development. This demonstrates that the presence and availability of positive male nurturance is not the exclusive domain of biological fathers.[24]

While grandfathers sometimes feel useless as caretakers, they are capable of making a unique and complementary contribution to parenting.[25] Grandfathers can help social, emotional, and cognitive development through physical play, sports, and encouraging achievement.[26] Research suggests that a warm and supportive relationship is the key to realizing the effects of the connection between an adult male and a child.[27] Just in case you still have doubts about the importance of men in child development, see the research findings summarized in Table 13.1.

Table 13.1. The Positive Effects of Relationships With Loving Male Adults: Grandfathers, Fathers, Stepfathers, and Mentors

Greater social engagement[a]	Greater self-esteem[f]
Turn-taking and appropriate ways of competing with others[b]	Appropriate risk-taking[g]
Improved sibling interactions[c]	Greater empathy[h]
Better social connection and social competency[d]	Fewer behavior problems[i]
Greater emotional security and psychological well-being[e]	Enhanced cognitive functioning[j]
	Better academic performance[k]

Although the dissolution of the family can have a devastating impact on every child, the absence of the father may have a particularly negative impact on young boys. By extended absence or abandoning the family, a father can leave his son with a deep emptiness that becomes filled with anger, rage, and confusion. Perhaps the increase in fatherless households explains why, between 1972 and 2000, the percentage of young adults (18–24) voting in American presidential elections dropped from 47% to 23%. In a study from the late 1990s where students were asked to name someone in their life whom they found to be inspiring—someone they considered a personal hero—the most common response was "no one."[28]

Despite good intentions, women cannot initiate boys into the world of men. Many men of my generation suffered abandonment by their fathers and tried to learn how to become men under their mothers' tutelage. Most of us entered adulthood knowing how not to be like our fathers but with few positive role models. Younger men need to be seen, admired, and guided by older men, just as older men need to be looked up to by younger men. When children continually shout, "Look at me, look at me," they are asking for exactly what they need—to be looked at with affection, pride, and admiration. Societal changes have led to the alienation of the generations and separated fathers from sons with unfortunate consequences.

Sequestering older adults in retirement communities and nursing homes is not only damaging to them but cuts off a natural social resource. If society deems that men over 65 are ridiculous relics of a bygone era and if older men buy into this role, they will not have the confidence and power to guide younger men into adulthood. Society as a whole will suffer the consequences of future generations of disconnected and disoriented men.

Fortunately, a wide array of older men can play an important role in the lives of young men. Teachers, coaches, uncles, and other older men can play a major role in the lives of younger men, especially when they take an interest in the nurturance of their minds and spirits. Boys need male role models to teach them how to be men. They need help to learn to use their strength for their own good and the good of the community. If this energy isn't guided, the resulting anger can be channeled into destructive antisocial behavior.

Younger men will always have greater physical and technological prowess than older men. Older men have the advantages of experience and wisdom. Together they have traditionally been the head and hands of the tribe; separated, they are disjoined and ineffectual, and their survival becomes tenuous. Wisdom is needed to guide the power and emotions of younger men, and fathers and grandfathers betray young men when they abdicate this responsibility.

The absence of the father, through either abandonment, preoccupation, or emotional distance, is experienced by the child as a betrayal not only by the father, but by the world, fate, and God. If you are a young man, find an older man and let him know you need his company, attention, and advice. If you are an older man, look for a young man to admire and spend time with. Your relationship might fire your minds, enliven your brains, and fill your hearts.

LISTENING WITH YOUR HEART

> *Perfect love sometimes does not come until the*
> *first grandchild.*
>
> *Welsh proverb*

Our ears translate mechanical vibrations into electrochemical signals that our brains convert into words and meanings. But sounds and words are only a small part of listening. Far more information is contained in the gestures and emotions that go along with what is being said. As we grow older, we have a better idea of other people's struggles because there is a good chance we've experienced them ourselves. As we age, we often grow more skilled in hearing the human struggle behind the surface conflicts. We also know that it's easier to accept support and advice when they are provided by someone who listens and shares in our feelings. Listening with your heart requires emotional presence and empathic attunement—it is wisdom in action.

Tim, a married man in his mid-30s, came to see me for help in dealing with stress. "I'm trying to be a good father to my three kids," he said, "but I always feel like I'm messing up. I say the wrong thing, get angry, or forget something that's important to them. I feel like I'm always apologizing." One day I asked him, "Do you know any men who you think are good fathers?" In reply, he told me a story about his own father:

> This memory begins with the typical smells and sounds of Thanksgiving Day. The combined aroma of turkey, dill, sage, cranberries, sweet potatoes. . . . You know that smell. My wife is rattling around in the kitchen searching for the serving platters. My daughters and son are playing board games in the den with my parents. The kids always get very excited when my folks come for a visit. They want attention from both of them at the same time, jockey for who will sit next to them, and pay rapt atten-

tion when they tell stories, especially the ones about the less stellar moments from my childhood. At this time, the kids were between 6 and 10, and I remember I was jealous of the attention they showed my folks, especially my dad. He seemed to be so good with them, so present, so tuned in.

While I was happy to see them getting along so well, I couldn't help but think about how absent he was when I was young. When I did see him, he was tired, irritable, distracted, and no fun to be with. He was always asking me questions or telling me what to do. "Did you do your homework? Did you brush your teeth? Did you clean your room?" He never asked me anything about what was happening with me. As I got older, I remember trying to stay out of his way by making plans with friends or working on projects in the garage. I would do anything to avoid his attitudes, his moods, and that annoyed look of his. So while I was happy for my kids, there was this underlying feeling of anger and resentment: "They are getting what I didn't get and now I have to be the heavy to make sure they do their homework. It's just not fair."

Somehow we negotiated Thanksgiving dinner and spent the afternoon hanging out in the backyard. At some point the badminton net went up, sides had been chosen, and we were all playing. My son Jimmy was on the same team with his mom and sisters and was getting riled up about not getting enough turns. Because he was the short-est, they could hit the birdie back over the net before it reached him. Fueling his frustration seemed to become the most entertaining part of the game for his sisters.

It was funny to watch them hit the birdie before it got to him, but they were taking it too far. Jimmy was aware that we were laughing at him, and he started to look hurt and angry. I was about to tell him to join our team when his anger got the best of him. "Shit!" came out of my innocent little boy's mouth; then I heard a loud thwack as he clubbed his sister with his racket, followed by a bloodcurdling yell. Then all hell broke loose. My wife screamed, "Jimmy!" My other daughter screamed, "She's bleeding!" And in her best Piglet voice, my mother added, "Oh dear. Oh dear me."

Something about blood calms my wife and activates her nursing skills. Jenny's bleeding head and its female entourage headed off to the bathroom, leaving three generations of males standing at the scene of the crime. I was feeling a lot of different emotions. I was worried about my daughter, I was angry at Jimmy, and I was ashamed that my father could see what a lousy father I had turned out to be. In the split second before the urge to smack Jimmy got the better of me, my dad stepped between us and put his arm around Jimmy's shoulder. Dad said, "Come and sit with me," and led Jimmy over to the bench.

My dad put his hand on Jimmy's knee. "It must have been really frustrating for you that they wouldn't let you hit the birdie; even worse, everyone laughed at you." Jimmy's rigid posture began to soften as his eyes welled with tears. Dad began to gently rub Jimmy's back as he melted into his lap. Jimmy sobbed for a while as his grandfather held him.

After a while my Dad said, "From time to time, everyone gets treated unfairly or gets made fun of. It's how you act at those difficult times that shows what you're made of. Remember last Fourth of July when I fell in the pool with my clothes on?" Jimmy's head started to shake, betraying his muffled laughter. Soon the three of us were laughing out loud. "You two guys laughed your butts off while I was bobbing up and down fishing for my shoe."

After awhile Jimmy looked at him thoughtfully and said, "And you didn't hit anybody on the head either. You just took it and smiled. It wasn't right what they did to me, but hitting Jenny really wasn't right." After a few moments he added, "I'm gonna go and tell her I'm sorry and then go to my room." Dad and I watched as Jimmy disappeared through the back door.

I thought back to my impulse to slap Jimmy. He would have been stunned and hurt, angry at me for adding to his pain and insult. If I had hit him, he would have run off to his room. I would have had to chase him down and order him to apologize to his sister and the entire family. It would have taken days for us to get close again and for the tension in the family to die down. I looked over to my dad, expecting "the look." Instead he smiled at me and said, "Quite a boy you have there. You've done a great job with him."

I was stunned! Not only had my father gently attained
the result that I would have bullied Jimmy into, but he was
complimenting me on being a good father! I felt like yell-
ing and crying at the same time. "How did you do that?"
I asked. "Do what?" Dad asked. "Get him to think about
what happened and apologize to his sister," I replied.

"Well, I could see that Jimmy was hurt, and I knew
why he did what he did. I could also see that he was scared
about what would happen next—what you would do and
how he should feel. He was angry and ashamed and would
have only felt worse if we came down on him. He needed
to have his feelings acknowledged before he could think
about his sister's and see the right thing to do. Once he felt
seen, he was able to do the right thing, just like you taught
him." I couldn't believe how wise my dad had gotten.

"Where did you learn that and why didn't you do it
that way when I was a kid?" "When I was your age," Dad
said, "I was all full of piss and vinegar and thought that
everything could be controlled through force. That's how
I made it through the war. That's how I built the business.
That's how I survived day to day. But as I've grown older,
I've had to learn some new ways of dealing with life. Like
an old pitcher, I have to rely on finesse instead of my fast-
ball; I've had to learn how to listen and pay attention to
other people's feelings and work from there.

"I know that I used to swat you and your brothers
and then tell you that you should never hit other people. I

can see now how crazy that is, doing one thing and trying to teach the opposite. Kids learn to treat others by how you treat them. I wish I would have known these things when you were young; I would have done things differently. You're a lot smarter than I was at your age, and I don't think it will take you as long to figure them out." That was the day I realized I still had a lot more to learn from my old man.

Optimal Challenge and Maximum Inclusion

If I were running in the stadium, ought I to
slacken my pace when approaching the goal?
Ought I not rather to put on speed?

—Diogenes

As an introspective child growing up in a blue-collar Catholic neighborhood, my curiosity and self-reflective nature were cause for suspicion. More than one concerned relative warned my mother to keep a careful eye on me. By my early teens, these musings evolved into a typical adolescent search for truth and my own identity, which led me to explore the world of lower Manhattan. Surrounded by the hippie culture of the late 1960s, I wandered through Greenwich Village, absorbing the sights and sounds of what I was told was a cultural revolution.

On one of these trips I discovered something unheard of in my neighborhood—vast used bookstores. Walking down the aisles of these dusty cathedrals, I marveled at the miles of sagging and overburdened shelves and imagined that truth must be hidden somewhere in one of these books. In contrast to the chaotic and youthful world of the streets, the folks inside these walls were seemingly at peace. They were perched on benches and leaned against walls, absorbed in thought, moving only to scratch an itch or turn a page. For some reason, I felt as if I had returned home for the first time.

My favorite bookshops came to be routine stops, and eventually the primary reason for my journeys to the city. I didn't have much money, so finding an interesting book usually meant staking out a corner and settling in for the afternoon. Over time, I became acquainted with some of the regulars, mostly immigrants from Eastern Europe. I became increasingly curious about them and looked for opportunities to strike up conversations. As luck would have it, my curiosity was met with their desire to tell stories.

Despite their different nationalities, ethnicities, and occupations, they all shared a relentless love of learning. Over the years, they had taken classes at the YMCA or the New School for Social Research from the likes of John Dewey, Wilhelm Reich, Elie Wiesel, and Robert Frost. Most spent what little disposable income they had on tickets to the theater or opera. At their feet, I learned the political and intellectual history of the first half of the 20th century. They taught me about the idealism of the early Communist Party, described what it felt like to hear Enrico

Caruso sing, and recounted conversations with Pablo
Picasso while standing in line at the butcher shop. I listened as one story melted into another, all the while making mental notes of the books, plays, and pieces of music I
would search out at the library. Somehow, these people had
escaped the gossip of daily life that permeated my home.
They possessed a set of values and source of meaning that
I desperately longed for.

Two of the most memorable characters were a couple,
Josef and Sarah. I clearly remember the afternoon I asked
Josef about a number tattooed on his inner forearm. Sarah
pulled up her sleeve to show me a similar marking. That
was the day that I first learned about the Holocaust from
two people who had somehow survived Hitler's insanity.
Although it had been many years since they were held in the
camps, the pain and horror reflected in their eyes was still
palpable and quickly found its way into my body and soul.

Later, I was befriended—adopted—by a retired theology
professor who talked to me for hours on end about the history of religion and the many expressions of spirituality. He
would attack the bookstore aisles with me at heel, tearing
book after book from the shelves. Tossing them to me as
I struggled to keep pace, he would say, "You have to read
this, and this, and this," as I followed him to the counter. He
would pay for the books, hand me the bag, and say, "Come
back next week and tell me what you think." A priceless
mentorship that I will never forget.

In stark contrast to my experiences with my family and

neighbors, these wise elders validated and encouraged my love of learning. Through their kind attention, I learned that curiosity was not to be feared but cherished and nurtured. More importantly, I learned that there were other people in the world like myself. Although some of them had endured unfathomable suffering, they still held on to their passion for life, learning, and connection with others. Through their openness and generosity, I discovered the strength of the human spirit and began to discover my own inner strength.

The process of nurturance through sharing knowledge cascades across the generations, resonating in our spirits and souls until we die. Through my interactions with these wise elders, I somehow gained the confidence to stand up to external pressures and pursue my own passions. They passed on their courage and character, which inspired me to become a teacher and writer and to encourage others to follow their dreams.

SHARING OUR LIVES

> When we die, there are two things we can leave behind us: genes and memes.
>
> Richard Dawkins

Wise elders are storytellers. They use the evocative potency of their tales to create a state of mind in listeners that maximizes receptivity and remembrance. The sacred space created by the storyteller nurtures the development of the youngster and completes the elder—over, and over, and over again. I believe that the combination of emotional and cognitive intelligence embodied within the storyteller is a way in which information and wisdom have been transmitted throughout time and across untold generations. As we age, the maturation of our brains maximizes our storytelling abilities, and we are driven to implant our stories into young minds, just as, earlier in life, we were driven to pass on our genes.

Stories serve us in many ways. They give form to the inchoate series of momentary experiences we confront each day. Our stories bring the past and future into the present moment and can serve as blueprints for working toward our goals. They also support a coherent sense of identity, as we become the protagonists of the stories we continually write and rewrite about ourselves. And, as we have seen, by combining a storyline with feelings, narratives support and enhance the all too fragile integration of our left and right cerebral hemispheres. Without narratives, I suspect that we would often be overwhelmed and confused by moment-to-moment experience.

The moral of a story, the lesson intended to be taken from the tale, supports our morale—the experience of confidence, hope, and enthusiasm with which we take on a challenge. Morale is most often used in describing combat troops who must keep their spirits up in the face of death, but it also applies to children who feel lost in a world that they don't understand. Many of life's challenges can be demoralizing, and stories can "remoralize" us by connecting us with others, sharing emotions, and inspiring us to be more like the heroes of our stories who have overcome life's challenges.[1] Positive stories provide direction, purpose, and the tenacity to persevere in the face of trouble.

Through the millennia of human history, narratives, songs, and rituals have been transmitted by elders to the young of the tribe. In the face of rapid cultural and technological changes, these stories and the moral teachings contained within them are getting lost, as is the morale they once supported. Yet the young continue to forage for meaningful narratives and now discover them in movies. Some contain the moral lessons of traditional narratives (e.g., *Star Wars, The Lord of the Rings, Harry Potter*), while many others reflect and reinforce fear and anxiety (e.g., *Friday the Thirteenth, The Living Dead*) that stories have traditionally been used to counterbalance. These violent and bloody narratives along with the evening news do not build morale but instead offer more evidence of a hostile and frightening world.

Thinking back once again to our list of wise people, we see that these individuals were not simply storytellers. They actually edited the narrative of human existence in ways that redefined how people relate to one another. Why is Oprah Winfrey in the company of Christ and Socrates on our list of wise people? I suspect it is precisely because of her ongoing mission to confront aspects of human suffering (e.g., child abuse, prejudice, eating disorders) that have been considered taboo. Her personal struggles in these areas make her all the more credible and worthy of respect. Uncommon among today's celebrities, Ms. Winfrey has gained her fame through a combination of business acumen and humility.

Throughout history, narratives told by elders were a primary means of transmitting knowledge and perpetuating culture. Over the last few millennia, our brains have changed little while society has changed a great deal. Elders still want to tell their stories, but few young people are listening. If elders surrender their position as storytellers, our children's children will be at the mercy of the highest bidder; Hollywood, fundamentalist megachurches, or radical cults, for their understanding of the world. If older adults abdicate their responsibilities as storytellers, we will remain in a state where young adults won't bother voting for president and when asked if they have a personal hero, they will answer "no one."[2]

WRITING OUR STORIES

Nothing that is worth doing can be achieved in a lifetime; therefore we must be saved by hope.

Reinhold Neibuhr

Creating a meaningful life story is a challenge at any age. Older adults, with more past than future, face a particular set of challenges. They ask themselves, "Have I used my time well? Have I accomplished what I had hoped to? Is there still something left that I want to do in order to complete my life?" Older adults depend as much as ever on the inclusiveness and coherence of their story for their sense of identity and emotional well-being.

Life can be seen as a series of stories we tell about ourselves, and as we age, these stories take on certain themes. One theme is the integration of loss—the loss of family, friends, physical abilities, and the places and times that only survive in our memories. These narratives are vital aspects of our ability to understand ourselves, grieve loss, and move on. Another theme is our emancipation from the unattainable and the unimportant. The powers of the body and the value of worldly accomplishments gradually move from center stage as the story of the self is rewritten around the heart and spirit. Just as in any good story, there needs to be an appreciation of the process—the victories and defeats, the loves and losses, and ultimately a sense of completion.

REVIEWING OUR LIVES

Life isn't about finding yourself. Life is about creating yourself.

George Bernard Shaw

Instead of an indication of diminished capacity, the rumination of older adults may reflect the struggle to make sense of their lives.[3] In response to this challenge, forms of therapy such as *life review therapy* have emerged to assist older adults in telling their stories.[4] Originally proposed by Robert Butler, life review therapy was designed to support and enhance the naturally occurring process of reminiscence. Therapists participate in their clients' storytelling and self-analysis by providing structure and guidance.[5] An example of this might be highlighting how a client has faced and overcome past challenges or asking about experiences that are not spontaneously brought forth. The underlying purpose of this guidance is to organize past narratives in a manner that supports current functioning and boosts the client's sense of confidence and efficacy.[6]

Life review can be carried out in individual or group settings and usually takes about a dozen sessions.[7] Themes such as life transitions and changing roles within the family are often addressed, as are experiences related to work, health, turning points, life values, and existential issues.[8] Participants are invited to bring scrapbooks, photographs, memorabilia, genealogies, and other objects to stimulate their memories.[9] As memories are evoked, telling stories and the input of the therapist become the matrix for constructing memory and meaning. Typical life review questions include the following:

- What happened to you during this time of your life?
- Can you give me a detailed picture of your experience?
- How did you feel at these moments?
- Did this event bring forward new aspects of your self?
- What did you learn about yourself during that time?
- How did you learn to cope with a specific loss?

- Did you receive any consolation from others?
- Did the events result in any personal insights?

Through the examination and evaluation of the content of their memories, clients are able to restructure their thinking about their experiences and reshape their ideas about their own identity. This process can aid in integrating memories of their past into here-and-now awareness, making them applicable to current concerns and conflicts. Reviewing past experiences when difficulties were faced and successfully overcome can provide both confidence and strategies for facing challenges in the present. The exploration, deconstruction, and reintegration of memory can result in building more cohesive and meaningful narratives. Some sample prompts for life review include:

- You've told me about what happened, but can you tell me how you felt about it?
- How do you feel about it now?
- Have you discovered any new meanings in these past experiences?
- How have these experiences contributed to the person you are today?
- What were your goals in life as a child, as a young adult, now?
- What do you hope to achieve in the future?
- What do you think your legacy will be?

Life review therapy is a nonthreatening, patient-driven intervention, appropriate for use with all older people, especially those who are resistant to psychotherapy.[10] As Hausman stated, "As events are thought out anew and are seen as part of an overall picture, they begin to assume a new and more comforting order."[11] This sence of order can help older adults maintain their identity, stability, and integrity during the later stages of life. Life review therapy has been shown to result in improved cognitive functioning, mood, and self-esteem.[12]

REMEMBERING HOW TO REMEMBER

It is never too late to be what we might have been.

George Eliot

The fact that human memory evolved in the context of storytelling is reflected in our memory abilities. Although we can hold only five to ten bits of new information in mind at any one time, we are able to remember and access a seemingly limitless number of stories and songs. And while older adults may have very detailed memories for experiences from decades ago, the difficulty we have in new learning points to the fact that our multiple systems of memory have different strengths, vulnerabilities, and patterns of aging.

As we've discussed, declines in explicit memory for new information are natural, but we do much better if we put disparate facts into a story. Most of us have seen this strategy in action in the extreme when memory experts remember hundreds of objects or people's names by creating a story in which the specific bits of information are placed. In essence, mnemonic techniques take information usually stored in low-capacity memory systems for discrete facts and store it in the much more powerful narrative memory networks. This strategy allows memory experts nearly infinite recall.

This is not a parlor trick; mnemonic techniques such as these have been shown to improve memory performance in people of all ages—including older adults.[13] In one memory training study, older adults used an imaginary trip to the tourist sites around Sydney harbor to enhance their memory for specific activities and events. The memory enhancement techniques that have proven successful with older adults may also enhance hippocampal functioning and support flagging prefrontal attentional mechanisms.[14]

Although many types of memory enhancement techniques have proven effective, research has been focusing on what is called multifactorial memory training. This approach combines education about aging and memory loss, relaxation training, and memory skills training.[15] These broad-based programs teach memory skills in the context of support and education, taking into account that pessimistic beliefs about aging and memory can increase anxiety, decrease motivation, and have a negative impact on all aspects of cognition.

A newer trend in memory training focuses on the benefit of group-based interventions. Several studies have shown these groups to improve attitudes and beliefs about personal memory while giving participants an increased sense of self-efficacy.[16] In a fascinating study, adults ages 65 to 82 were trained in acting techniques, followed by rehearsals and the performance of a theatrical scene.[17] Although the training was in no way targeted to memory, participants had significantly higher memory scores after these acting exercises. The cognitive challenge of learning lines coupled with the physical activity were thought to be supportive of new learning.[18]

Although the researchers primarily attributed the participants' improved memory to the mental effort involved in learning and performing the role, I wonder if the participants' social and emotional involvement in this enterprise may not have been just as important. The authors gave some credence to the role of social factors near the conclusion of their work:

> Undoubtedly, the facilitative effects of socializing were also involved; the experimenters frequently observed the participants playfully interacting with one another during breaks, openly revealing their feelings in the same way that their assigned characters did during the play. Thus, theatrical training involves not only cognitive factors, but emotive, social, and physiological ones as well.[19]

The fact that social interaction can create an atmosphere that enhances self-esteem and memory performance harkens back to the evolutionary foundation of memory as an interactive process of storytelling. Mutual support, encouragement, positive personal engagements, and getting up and moving around, in and of themselves, activate biochemical processes that enhance protein synthesis, brain growth, and new learning.

HELPER'S HIGH

If you forget who you are, serve someone else until it comes to you.

Anonymous

For almost everyone, helping others feels good. Of 1,500 female volunteers, 88% reported a pleasurable physical sensation in reaction to helping others. They alternately described the feeling as a high, a warm feeling, a sense of increased energy, or some combination of all three.[20] These sensations are akin to those we experience during exercise or when we fall in love and only occur when we are face-to-face with those to whom we are giving. Mailing checks to your favorite charities is a good thing to do, but it likely doesn't activate the same biochemical processes.

Older adults who volunteered to give massages to infants demonstrated lower postmassage levels of stress hormones and an enhancement of immunological biochemistry.[21] Even witnessing the altruistic behavior of others can boost our immune systems, as demonstrated by an increase in protective antibodies in subjects after watching a film about Mother Theresa caring for the poor in Calcutta.[22]

As in so many other instances, it appears that nature reinforces human connectedness by utilizing the same oxytocin, endorphin, and dopamine systems it employs for bonding and attachment. And because higher levels of these chemicals correlate with well-being and enhanced immunological functioning, altruism can be good for your health. This has been shown in a number of studies where altruism and volunteering correlate with indicators of physical and emotional health. Altruistic and caring acts correlate with lower levels of stress, anxiety, depression, and hopelessness and a greater sense of well-being. They also support increased immunological functioning, greater health, and less pain from a variety of illnesses.

This is all good news for older adults! According to the 2000 U.S. Census, 42% of 65- to 74-year-olds and 26.6% of those over 75 volunteer their time to a wide array of community services and activities. The number of hours that older adults volunteer each year is almost double (96 vs. 52) the national average for all ages.[23] This indicates that older adults are naturally drawn to generative and altruistic behavior and are well aware of the benefits they receive by giving. Typical older volunteer are individuals who value the welfare of others, spend their own money in order to be of service, and display psychological well-being.[24] Furthermore, they have higher self-esteem and a healthy sense of social integration.

Volunteering has long been associated with positive psychological effects, a higher degree of life satisfaction, and decreased levels of depression and anxiety.[25] Studies have also suggested that providing social support and volunteering reduces the risk of mortality.[26] So why does altruism have a positive effect on longevity? The social reasons include a sense of structure, purpose, and expanded social networks. Other reasons related to self-efficacy include feeling useful, increased self-esteem, and enhanced self-identity. Providing support to others was shown to reduce the risk of mortality in a sample of 1,532 older married adults.

So if you want to live a longer and healthier life, put in some time volunteering in your community as soon as you can. Start by contacting organizations such as Senior Corps, Retired and Senior Volunteer Corp (RSVP), or Service Corps of Retired Executives (SCORE). If you decide to "unretire" or want to learn new skills, contact SeniorNet, ReServe, or Experience Works to explore ideas for career opportunities. If this sounds too involved or more than you are interested in, go to your local library and volunteer to read to children. You may even want to slip in some stories of your own while you're at it.

EXPECTATION IS DESTINY

My father planted for me, and I planted for my children.
Hebrew Proverb

Although all animals have an instinct to live, humans also need a reason. The themes of optimal challenge and maximum inclusion need to be embedded within a set of ideas that lead us to maintain healthy brains. In fact, Okinawan centenarians attribute their unusually long life spans to having *ikigai*—a purpose for living. When older adults are respected, depended upon, and needed, most respond in a positive and life-affirming way that benefits all generations. The isolation and exclusion of older adults is a great tragedy for them, our children, and ourselves.

We lose many people on the way to old age. Grandparents, parents, beloved mentors and teachers, friends and lovers, sometimes even our children leave us behind. The experience of loss is as natural as our continued need for attachments. Maintaining an openness to making new attachments and finding new sources of meaning is important for a vital life. Instead of becoming the sum of all we have lost, we have to continue to learn, love, and keep our eyes on the horizon.

It's clear that our brains are organs of adaptation, embedded in a body, and fundamentally social in nature. In order to maximize the brain's functioning, we require proper physical, intellectual, and interpersonal stimulation. This means that everyone at every age should be encouraged to be active, engaged, and challenged to the limits of their capabilities. Our brains need to receive the message that adaptation is still necessary and that neural growth is still required.

The predictors of sustained cognitive health, such as

education, intellectual stimulation, and a sense of self-efficacy, all point to the importance of continuing to take on challenges, reduce stress where possible, and enjoy living and loving. After decades of exploring mental health throughout the life span, George Vaillant suggested that those who stay most vital and alive are those who are capable of learning from the next generation.[28] He added that these are the same people who are best able to care for their children, grandchildren, and other younger people. This is a wonderfully human description of both the miracle of ongoing neural plasticity and the process of becoming a wise elder.

From the perspective of social neuroscience, full retirement may be inappropriate for many of us, just as full-time employment may not be in the best interest of parents with young children. A MacArthur Foundation study of aging suggested that older and younger adults learn to share jobs so that each could work half days and cover for the other when fatigue or emergencies arise. Older workers could mentor younger ones, while younger workers could help their elders keep abreast of newer technical developments. More flexible employment programs could also allow a series of steps on the way toward full retirement that would continue to keep older adults challenged to the limits of their changing capabilities.

Another potential solution to elder isolation communities called NORCs (naturally occurring retirement communities). These are organizations of elders who want to remain in their homes but require one or more support services in order to do so. NORC members receive discounts on everything from in-home care to medication management as well as access to free exercise classes and walking groups. The contact and support that emerge from these organizations create a social network that works against isolation and the types of problems that lead elders to lose their independence and become institutionalized.

Another wonderful idea is to combine retirement developments and nursing homes with nurseries, day care centers, and preschools to allow older adults to participate in child care. This has practical as well as emotional benefits for everyone involved and is already occurring in some retirement communities associated with universities, such as the Kendal community at Oberlin College. One foster care facility in California created a living situation where children and senior citizens share land and resources. Although no formal agreement was established about the children and older adults interacting, they gradually became interwoven into each other's lives. One former gang member adopted a frail senior, checked in on her regularly, and helped her with difficult chores. Another couple became so attached to a young basketball player that they attended each of his games throughout the season. The success of this program has been reflected in the improved well-being of both the children and adult participants.

A LIFELONG MEDITATION

*Your sacred place is where you can find yourself again
and again.*

Joseph Campbell

Our ideas, beliefs, and myths about aging determine how we view others and ourselves. If we go through our lives with positive ideas about aging, we will have better memories, have better health, and live longer than those who have accepted negative stereotypes about aging.[29] Thus, our first order of business in creating and maintaining a healthy brain is to change our beliefs about what it means to age: creating narratives and images of a positive and participatory adulthood. The second is to work diligently to propagate these positive ideas throughout our culture and across the generations. My hope is that the ideas and feelings expressed within this book are a small step in the right direction, one of many steps still ahead of us.

Many years ago I spent an evening talking with a Zen priest at his monastery north of Mt. Fuji. As part of his religious training, he had spent 10 years slowly walking across Japan. This decade-long walk consisted of taking a step, ringing a bell, and saying a prayer. Through 40 seasons, a number of illnesses, and what sounded to me like occasional hallucinations, he continued to take a step, ring his bell, and say a prayer. As I tried to fathom the enormity of this amazing accomplishment, the obvious question struck me—Why?

What was the purpose of such an incredible act of will and self-denial? What could be so important? I struggled to think of a respectful way to ask such a brazen question. I finally asked, "Sensei, what was the goal of your act of discipline? What did you hope to accomplish?" Matter-of-factly, Sensei told me that it was a way to learn to pay attention to what was around him and to become less burdened by the prejudices of his mind. Amazed by the simplicity of his response, I clumsily asked, "But why so long?"

Without missing a beat, he replied, "Because that's how long it takes."

CREDITS

TABLE 3.1

a. Szinovacz, M. E., DeViney, S., & Atkinson, M. P. (1999). Effects of surrogate parenting on grandparents' well-being. *Journal of Gerontology: Social Sciences, 54B*, S376–S388.

b. Pruchno, R. A. (1999). Raising grandchildren: The experiences of black and white grandmothers. *Gerontologist, 39*, 209–221.

c. Baydar, N., & Brooks-Gunn, J. (1998). Profiles of grandmothers who help care for their grandchildren in the United States. *Family Relations, 47*, 385–393.

d. Waldrop, D. P., & Weber, J. A. (2001). From grandparent to caregiver: The stress and satisfaction of raising grandchildren. *Families in Society: The Journal of Contemporary Human Services, 5*, 461–472; Robertson, J. F. (1977). Grandmotherhood: A study of role conceptions. *Journal of Marriage and Family, 39*(1), 165–174.

e. Robertson, J. F. (1977). Grandmotherhood: A study of role conceptions. *Journal of Marriage and Family, 39*(1), 165–174.

f. Gattai, F. B., & Musatti, T. (1999). Grandmothers' involvement in grandchildren's care: Attitudes, feelings, and emotions. *Family Relations, 48*, 35–42; Reitzes, D. C., & Mutran, E. J. (2004). Grandparent identity, intergenerational family identity, and well-being. *Journal of Gerontology: Social Sciences, 59B*, S213–S219.

g. Pruchno, R. A. (1999). Raising grandchildren: The experiences of black and white grandmothers. *Gerontologist, 39*, 209–221.

h. Kropf, N. P., & Burnette, D. (2003). Grandparents as family caregivers: Lessons for intergenerational education. *Educational Gerontology, 29*, 361–372.

i. Burton, L. (1992). Black grandparents rearing children of drug-addicted parents: Stressors, outcomes, and social service needs. *Gerontologist, 32*, 744–751.

j. Hayslip, B., Jr., & Kaminski, P. L. (2005). Grandparents raising their grandchildren: A review of the literature and suggestions for practice. *Gerontologist, 45,* 262–269.

k. Gattai, F. B., & Musatti, T. (1999). Grandmothers' involvement in grandchildren's care: Attitudes, feelings, and emotions. *Family Relations, 48,* 35–42.

l. Szinovacz, M. E., & Davey, A. (2006). Effects of retirement and grandchild care on depressive symptoms. *International Journal of Aging and Human Development, 62,* 1–20.

m. Burton, L. (1992). Black grandparents rearing children of drug-addicted parents: Stressors, outcomes, and social service needs. *Gerontologist, 32,* 744–751; Jendrek, M. P. (1993). Grandparents who parent their grandchildren: Effects on lifestyle. *Journal of Marriage and the Family, 55,* 609–621.

n. Burton, L., & Devries, C. (1992). Challenges and rewards: African American grandparents as surrogate parents. *Generations, 16,* 51–54; Szinovacz, M. E., DeViney, S., & Atkinson, M. P. (1999). Effects of surrogate parenting on grandparents' well-being. *Journal of Gerontology: Social Sciences, 54B,* S376–S388; Gattai, F. B., & Musatti, T. (1999). Grandmothers' involvement in grandchildren's care: Attitudes, feelings, and emotions. *Family Relations, 48,* 35–42.

o. Szinovacz, M. E., & Davey, A. (2006). Effects of retirement and grandchild care on depressive symptoms. *International Journal of Aging and Human Development, 62,* 1–20; Jendrek, M. P. (1993). Grandparents who parent their grandchildren: Effects on lifestyle. *Journal of Marriage and the Family, 55,* 609–621.

p. Antonucci, T. C. (1990). Social supports and social relationships. In R. H. Binstock and L. K. George (Eds.), *Handbook of aging and the social sciences* (3rd ed., pp. 205–226). New York: Academic Press; Musil, C. M., & Ahmad, M. (2002). Health of grandmothers: A comparison by caregiver status. *Journal of Aging and Health, 14,* 96–121.

q. Neugarten, B. L., & Weinstein, K. K. (1964). The changing American grandparent. *Journal of Marriage and the Family, 26*(2), 199–204.

r. Pruchno, R. A. (1999). Raising grandchildren: The experiences of black and white grandmothers. *Gerontologist, 39,* 209–221.

s. Burton, L., & Devries, C. (1992). Challenges and rewards: African American grandparents as surrogate parents. *Generations, 16,* 51–54.

t. Peterson, C. C. (1999). Grandfathers' and grandmothers' satisfaction with the grandparenting role: Seeking new answers to old questions. *International Journal of Aging and Human Development, 49,* 61–78.

TABLE 5.1

a. Allen, J. S., Bruss, J., Brown, C. K., & Damasio, H. (2005). Normal neuroanatomical variation due to age: The major lobes and a parcellation of the temporal region. *Neurobiology of Aging, 26,* 1245–1260; Bartzokis, G., Beckson, M., Lu, P. H., Nuechterlein, K. H., Edwards, N., & Mintz, J. (2001). Age-related changes in frontal and temporal lobe volumes in men. *Archives of General Psychiatry, 58,* 461–465; Good, C. D., Johnsrude, I. S., Ashburner, J., Henson, R. D., Friston, K. J., & Frackowiak, R. S. (2001). Cerebral asymmetry and the effects of sex and handedness on brain structure: A voxel-based morphometric analysis of 465 normal adult human brains. *NeuroImage, 14*(3), 685–700; Grieve, S. M., Clark, C. R., Williams, L. M., Peduto, A. J., & Gordon, E. (2005). Preservation of limbic and paralimbic structures in aging. *Human Brain Mapping, 25,* 391–401; Jernigan, T. L., Archibald, S. L., Fennema-Notestine, C., Gamst, A. C., Stout, J. C., Bonner, J., et al. (2001). Effects of age on tissues and regions of the cerebrum and cerebellum. *Neurobiology of Aging, 22,* 581–594; Pfefferbaum, A., Mathalon, D. H., Sullivan, E. V., Rawles, J. M., Zipursky, R. B., & Lim, K. O. (1994). A quantitative magnetic resonance imaging study of changes in brain morphology from infancy to late adulthood. *Archives of Neuroscience, 51,* 874–887; Sowell, E. R., Peterson, B. S., Thompson, P. M., Welcome, S. E., Henkenius, A. L., & Toga, A. W. (2003). Mapping cortical change across the human life span. *Nature Neuroscience, 6,* 309–315; Tisserand, D. J., van Boxtel, M. P. J., Pruessner, J. C., Hofman, P., Evans, A. C., & Jolles, J. (2004). A voxel-based morphometric study to determine individual differences in gray matter density associated with age and cognitive change over time. *Cerebral Cortex, 14,* 966–973.

b. Sowell, E. R., Thompson, P. M., Tessner, K. D., & Toga, A. W. (2001). Mapping continued brain growth and gray matter density reduction in dorsal frontal cortex: Inverse relationships during postadolescent brain maturation. *Journal of Neuroscience, 21,* 8819–8829; Sowell, E. R., Trauner, D. A., Gamst, A., & Jernigan, T. L. (2002). Development of cortical and subcortical brain structures in childhood and adolescence: A structural MRI study. *Developmental Medicine & Child Neurology, 44,* 4–16.

c. Good, C. D., Johnsrude, I. S., Ashburner, J., Henson, R. D., Friston, K. J., & Frackowiak, R. S. (2001). Cerebral asymmetry and the effects of sex and handedness on brain structure: A voxel-based morphometric analysis of 465 normal adult human brains. *NeuroImage, 14*(3), 685–700.

d. Bartzokis, G., Beckson, M., Lu, P. H., Nuechterlein, K. H., Edwards, N., & Mintz, J. (2001). Age-related changes in frontal and temporal lobe volumes in men. *Archives of General Psychiatry, 58*, 461–465; Bartzokis, G., Sultzer, P., & Lu, P. H. (2004). Heterogeneous age-related breakdown of white matter structural integrity: Implications for cortical "disconnection" in aging and Alzheimer's disease. *Neurobiology of Aging, 25*, 843–851; Davatzikos, C., & Resnick, S. M. (2002). Degenerative age changes in white matter connectivity visualized in vivo using magnetic resonance imaging. *Cerebral Cortex, 12*, 767–771; Nusbaum, A. O., Tang, C. Y., Buchsbaum, M. S., Wei, T. C., & Atlas, S. W. (2001). Regional and global changes in cerebral diffusion with normal aging. *American Journal of Neuroradiology, 22*, 136–142; O'Sullivan, M., Jones, D. K., Summers, P. E., Morris, R. G., Williams, S. C. R., & Markus, H. S. (2001). Evidence for cortical "disconnection" as a mechanism of age-related cognitive decline. *Neurology, 57*, 632–638; Salat, D. H., Tuch, D. S., Greve, D. N., van der Kouwe, A. J. W., Hevelone, N. D., Zaleta, A. K., et al. (2005). Age-related alterations in white matter microstructure measured by diffusion tensor imaging. *Neurobiology of Aging, 26*, 1215–1227; Sowell, E. R., Peterson, B. S., Thompson, P. M., Welcome, S. E., Henkenius, A. L., & Toga, A. W. (2003). Mapping cortical change across the human life span. *Nature Neuroscience, 6*, 309–315; Grieve, S. M., Clark, C. R., Williams, L. M., Peduto, A. J., & Gordon, E. (2005). Preservation of limbic and paralimbic structures in aging. *Human Brain Mapping, 25*, 391–401; Resnick, S. M., Goldszal, A. F., Davatzikos, C., Golski, S., Kraut, M. A., Metter, E. J., et al. (2000). One-year age changes in MRI brain volumes in older adults. *Cerebral Cortex, 10*, 464–472; Guttman, C. R. G., Jolesz, F. A., Kikinis, R., Killiany, R. J., Moss, M. B., Sandor, T., et al. (1998). White matter changes with normal aging. *Neurology, 50*, 972–978; Pfefferbaum, A., Adalsteinsson, E., & Sullivan, E. V. (2005). Frontal circuitry degradation marks healthy adult aging: Evidence from diffusion tensor imaging. *NeuroImage, 26*, 891–899; Pfefferbaum, A., Mathalon, D. H., Sullivan, E. V., Rawles, J. M., Zipursky, R. B., & Lim, K. O. (1994). A quantitative magnetic resonance imaging study of changes in brain morphology from infancy to late adulthood. *Archives of Neuroscience, 51*, 874–887; Pfefferbaum, A., Sullivan, E. V., Hedehus, M., Lim, K. O., Adalsteinsson, E., & Moseley, M. (2000). Age-related decline in brain white matter anisotropy measured with spatially corrected echoplanar diffusion tensor imaging. *Magnetic Resonance in Medicine, 44*, 259–268; Wahlund, L.-O., Almkvist, O., Basun, H., & Julin, P. (1996).

MRI in successful aging, a 5-year follow-up study from the eighth to ninth decade of life. *Magnetic Resonance Imaging, 14,* 601–608.

TABLE 7.2

a. Labouvie-Vief, G. (1990). Wisdom as integrated thought: Historical and developmental perspectives. In R. J. Sternberg (Ed.), *Wisdom: Its nature, origins, and development* (pp. 52–83). New York: Cambridge University Press.

TABLE 7.3

a. Erikson, E. H., (1982). *The life cycle completed: A review.* New York: Norton.

TABLE 7.4

a. Vaillant, G. E. (2002). *Aging well.* New York: Little, Brown and Company.

TABLE 7.5

a. Cohen, G. D. (2005). *The mature mind: The positive power of the aging brain.* New York: Basic Books.

TABLE 11.1

a. Galli, R. L., Shukitt-Hale, B., Youdim, K. A., & Joseph, J. A. (2002). Fruit polyphenolics and brain aging: Nutritional interventions targeting age-related neuronal and behavioral deficits. *Annals of the New York Academy of Sciences, 959,* 128–132; Lau, F. C., Bielinski, D. F., & Joseph J. A. (2007). Inhibitory effects of blueberry extract on the production of inflammatory mediators in lipopolysaccharide-activated BV2 microglia. *Journal of Neuroscience Research, 85*(5), 1010–1017; Lau, F. C., Shukitt-Hale, & Joseph, J. A. (2005). The beneficial effects of fruit polyphenols on brain aging. *Neurobiology of Aging 268,* S128–S132.

b. Duthie, S. J., Whalley, L. J., Collins, A. R., Leaper, S., Berger, K., & Deary, I. J. (2002). Homocysteine, b vitamin status, and cognitive function in the elderly. *The American Journal of Clinical Nutrition, 75,* 908–913; Kruman, I. I., Kumaravel, T. S., Lohani, A., Pedersen, W. A., Cutler, R. G., Kruman, Y., Haughey, N., Lee, J., Evans, M., & Mattson, M. P. (2002). Folic acid deficiency and homocysteine impair DNA repair in hippocampal neurons and sensitize them to amyloid toxicity in experimental models of alzheimer's disease. *Journal of Neuroscience, 22*(5), 1752–1762; Mattson, M. P. (2003). Gene-diet interactions in brain

aging and neurodegenerative disorders. *Annals of Internal Medicine,*
139(5), 441–444; Mattson, M. P., Kruman, I. I., &Duan, W. (2002).
Folic acid and homocysteine in age-related disease. *Ageing Research*
Reviews, 1, 95–111.

c. Uauy, R. & Dangour, A. D. (2006). Nutrition in brain development and
aging: role of essential fatty acids. *Nutrition Reviews, 64*(5), S24–S33.

d. Franco, O. H., Burger, H., Lebrun, C. E. I., Peeters, P. H. M., Lamberts,
S. W. J., Grobbee, D. E., et al. (2005). Higher dietary intake of lignans
is associated with better cognitive performance in postmenopausal
women. *The Journal of Nutrition, 135,* 1190–1195; Zhao, L., Chen, Q.,
Brinton, R. D. (2002). Neuroprotective and neurotrophic efficacy of
phytoestrogens in cultured hippocampal neurons. *Experimental Biology*
and Medicine, 22(7), 509–519.

TABLE 11.2

a. Wolkove, N., Elkholy, O., Baltzan, M., & Palayew, M. (2007). Sleep
and aging: 2. Management of sleep disorders in older people. *Canadian*
Medical Association Journal, 176(10), 1449–1454.

TABLE 12.1

a. Cacioppo, J. T., & Berntson, G. G. (2002). Social neuroscience. In J. T.
Cacioppo, G. G. Berntson, R. Adolphs, C. S. Carter, R. J. Davidson,
M. McClintock, et al. (Eds.) *Foundations in social neuroscience* (pp.3–10).
Cambridge, MA: MIT Press; Uchino, B. N., Cacioppo, J. T., & Kiecolt-
Glaser, J. K. (1996). The relationship between social support and physi-
ological processes: A review with emphasis on underlying mechanisms
and implications for health. *Psychological Bulletin, 119*(3), 488–531.

b. Cacioppo, J. T., & Berntson, G. G. (2002). Social neuroscience. In J. T.
Cacioppo, G. G. Berntson, R. Adolphs, C. S. Carter, R. J. Davidson,
M. McClintock, et al. (Eds.) *Foundations in social neuroscience* (pp.3–10).
Cambridge, MA: MIT Press; Hanson, B. S., Isacsson, S.-O., Janzon,
L., Lindell, S.-E., & Rastam, L. (1988). Social anchorage and blood
pressure in elderly men—A population study. *Journal of Hypertension,*
6, 503–510; Kamarck, T. W., Manuck, S. B., & Jennings, J. R. (1990).
Social support reduces cardiovascular reactivity to psychological chal-
lenge: A laboratory model. *Psychosomatic Medicine, 52,* 42–58.

c. Thomas, P. D., Goodwin, J. M., & Goodwin, J. S. (1985). Effect of
social support on stress-related changes in cholesterol level, uric acid
level, and immune function in an elderly sample. *American Journal of*
Psychiatry, 142, 735–737.

2

Credits

271

d. Lepore, S. J., Allen, K. A. M., & Evans, G. W. (1993). Social support lowers cardiovascular reactivity to an acute stressor. *Psychosomatic Medicine, 55,* 518–524.

e. Eng, P. M., Rimm, E. B., Fitzmaurice, G., & Kawachi, I. (2002). Social ties and change in social ties in relation to subsequent total and cause-specific mortality and coronary heart disease incidence in men. *American Journal of Epidemiology, 155,* 700–709; Orth-Gomér, K., Rosengren, A., & Wilhelmsen, L. (1993). Lack of social support and incidence of coronary heart disease in middle-aged Swedish men. *Psychosomatic Medicine, 55,* 37–43.

f. Berkman, L. F. (1995). The role of social relations in health promotion. *Psychosomatic Medicine, 57,* 245–254; Seeman, T. (1996). Social ties and health: The benefits of social integration. *Annals of Epidemiology, 6,* 442–451.

g. Cohen, S. (2004). Social relationships and health. *American Psychologist, 59676*–684; Cohen, S., Doyle, W. J., Turner, R., Alper, C. M., & Skoner, D. P. (2003). Sociability and susceptibility to the common cold. *Psychological Science, 14*(5), 389–395; House, J. S., Landis, K. R., & Umberson, D. (1988). Social relationships and health. *Science, 241*(4865), 540–545; Kiecolt-Glaser, J. K., McGuire, L., Robles, T. F., & Glaser, R. (2002). Psychoneuroimmunology and psychosomatic medicine: Back to the future. *Psychosomatic Medicine, 64,* 15–28; Seeman, T. (1996). Social ties and health: The benefits of social integration. *Annals of Epidemiology, 6,* 442–451; Thomas, P. D., Goodwin, J. M., & Goodwin, J. S. (1985). Effect of social support on stress-related changes in cholesterol level, uric acid level, and immune function in an elderly sample. *American Journal of Psychiatry, 142,* 735–737; Uchino, B. N., Cacioppo, J. T., & Kiecolt-Glaser, J. K. (1996). The relationship between social support and physiological processes: A review with emphasis on underlying mechanisms and implications for health. *Psychological Bulletin, 119*(3), 488–531.

h. Cohen, S. (2004). Social relationships and health. *American Psychologist, 59676*–684; Cohen, S., Doyle, W. J., Turner, R., Alper, C. M., & Skoner, D. P. (2003). Sociability and susceptibility to the common cold. *Psychological Science, 14*(5), 389–395; House, J. S., Landis, K. R., & Umberson, D. (1988). Social relationships and health. *Science, 241*(4865), 540–545; Kiecolt-Glaser, J. K., McGuire, L., Robles, T. F., & Glaser, R. (2002). Psychoneuroimmunology and psychosomatic medicine: Back to the future. *Psychosomatic Medicine, 64,* 15–28; Seeman, T. (1996). Social ties and health: The benefits of social integration. *Annals of Epidemiology, 6,* 442–451; Thomas, P. D., Goodwin, J. M., & Goodwin, J. S. (1985). Effect of social support on stress-related changes in cholesterol level, uric acid level, and immune function in an elderly sample. *American Journal of Psychiatry, 142*, 735–737; Uchino, B. N., Cacioppo, J. T., & Kiecolt-Glaser, J. K. (1996). The relationship between social support and physiological processes: A review with emphasis on underlying mechanisms and implications for health. *Psychological Bulletin, 119*(3), 488–531.

i. Kiecolt-Glaser, J. K., Rickers, D., George, J., Messick, G., Speicher, C. E., Garner, W., et al. (1984). Urinary cortisol levels, cellular immunocompetency, and lonliness in psychiatric inpatients. *Psychosomatic Medicine, 46*(1), 15–23.

j. Cutrona, C., Russell, D., & Rose, J. (1986). Social support and adaptation to stress by the elderly. *Journal of Psychology and Aging, 1*, 47–54; Eng, P. M., Rimm, E. B., Fitzmaurice, G., & Kawachi, I. (2002). Social ties and change in social ties in relation to subsequent total and cause-specific mortality and coronary heart disease incidence in men. *American Journal of Epidemiology, 155*, 700–709; Larson, R. (1978). Thirty years of research on the subjective well-being of older Americans. *Journal of Gerontology, 33*, 109–125; Shye, D., Mullooly, J. P., Freeborn, D. K., & Pope, C. R. (1995). Gender differences in the relationship between social network support and mortality: A longitudinal study of an elderly cohort. *Social Science and Medicine, 41*, 935–947; Uchino, B. N., Cacioppo, J. T., & Kiecolt-Glaser, J. K. (1996). The relationship between social support and physiological processes: A review with emphasis on underlying mechanisms and implications for health. *Psychological Bulletin, 119*(3), 488–531.

k. Anson, O. (1989). Marital status and women's health revisited: The importance of a proximate adult. *Journal of Marriage and the Family, 51*, 185–194.

l. Cohen, S., Doyle, W. J., Turner, R., Alper, C. M., & Skoner, D. P. (2003). Sociability and susceptibility to the common cold. *Psychological Science, 14*(5), 389–395.

m. Cohen, S. (2004). Social relationships and health. *American Psychologist, 59*676–684.

n. Seeman, T. (1996). Social ties and health: The benefits of social integration. *Annals of Epidemiology, 6*, 442–451.

o. Kawachi, I., & Berkman, L. F. (2001). Social ties and mental health. *Journal of Urban Health, 78*(3), 458–467; Russell, D. W., & Cutrona, C. E. (1991). Social support, stress, and depressive symptoms among the elderly: Test of a process model. *Psychology and Aging, 6*, 190–201.

p. Cohen, S., Doyle, W. J., Turner, R., Alper, C. M., & Skoner, D. P.

(2003). Sociability and susceptibility to the common cold. *Psychological Science, 14*(5), 389–395.

q. Cohen, S. (2004). Social relationships and health. *American Psychologist, 59*676–684; Russell, D. W., & Cutrona, C. E. (1991). Social support, stress, and depressive symptoms among the elderly: Test of a process model. *Psychology and Aging, 6*, 190–201; Segrin, C. (2003). Age moderates the relationship between social support and psychosocial problems. *Human Communication Research, 29*(3), 317–342; Vandervoort, D. (1999). Quality of social support in mental and physical health. *Current Psychology, 18*(2), 205–222.

r. Siegel, J. M., & Kuykendall, D. H. (1990). Loss, widowhood, and psychological distress among the elderly. *Journal of Consulting and Clinical Psychology, 58*, 519–524.

s. Bassuk, S. S., Glass, T. A., & Berkman, L. F. (1999). Social disengagement and incident cognitive decline in community-dwelling elderly persons. *Annals of Internal Medicine, 131*, 165–173; Cohen, S. (2004). Social relationships and health. *American Psychologist, 59*676–684.

t. Cacioppo, J. T., & Berntson, G. G. (2002). Social neuroscience. In J. T. Cacioppo, G. G. Berntson, R. Adolphs, C. S. Carter, R. J. Davidson, M. McClintock, et al. (Eds.) *Foundations in social neuroscience* (pp.3–10). Cambridge, MA: MIT Press.

TABLE 13.1

a. Caldera, Y. M. (2004). Paternal involvement and infant-father attachment: A Q-Set study. *Fathering, 2*, 191–210.

b. DeKlyen, M., Speltz, M. L., & Greenberg, M. T. (1998). Fathering and early onset conduct problems: Positive and negative parenting, father-son attachment, and the marital context. *Clinical Child and Family Psychology Review, 1*, 3–21.

c. Volling, B. L., & Belsky, J. (1992). The contribution of mother-child and father-child relationships to the quality of sibling interaction: A longitudinal study. *Child Development, 63*, 1209–1222.

d. Harris, K. M., Furstenberg, F. F., Jr., & Marmer, J. K. (1998). Paternal involvement with adolescents in intact families: The influence of fathers over the life course. *Demography, 35*(2), 201–216; Lamb, M. E. (Ed.). (1997). *The role of the father in child development* (3rd ed.). New York: John Wiley & Sons; MacDonald, K., & Parke, R. D. (1984). Bridging the gap: Parent-child play interaction and peer interactive competence. *Child Development, 55*, 1265–1277; Ricks, S. S. (1985). Father-infant interactions: A review of empirical research. *Family Relations, 34*, 505–

511; Rosenberg, J., & Wilcox, W. B. (2006). *The importance of fathers in the healthy development of children.* Washington, DC: U. S. Department of Health and Human Services, Administration for Children and Families, Administration on Children, Youth and Families, Children's Bureau, Office on Child Abuse and Neglect.

e. Caldera, Y. M. (2004). Paternal involvement and infant-father attachment: A Q-Set study. *Fathering, 2,* 191–210; Dubowitz, H., Black, M. M., Cox, C. E., Kerr, M. A., Litrownik, A. J., Radhakrishna, A., et al. (2001). Father involvement and children's functioning at age 6 years: A multisite study. *Child Maltreatment, 6*(4), 300–309; Harris, K. M., Furstenberg, F. F., Jr., & Marmer, J. K. (1998). Paternal involvement with adolescents in intact families: The influence of fathers over the life course. *Demography, 35*(2), 201–216; Rosenberg, J., & Wilcox, W. B. (2006). *The importance of fathers in the healthy development of children.* Washington, DC: U. S. Department of Health and Human Services, Administration for Children and Families, Administration on Children, Youth and Families, Children's Bureau, Office on Child Abuse and Neglect.

f. Lamb, M. E. (Ed.). (1997). *The role of the father in child development* (3rd ed.). New York: John Wiley & Sons; Zimmerman, M. A., Salem, D. A., & Maton, K. I. (1995). Family structure and psychosocial correlates among urban African-American adolescent males. *Child Development, 66,* 1598–1613.

g. Kazura, K. (2000). Fathers' qualitative and quantitative involvement: An investigation of attachment, play, and social interactions. *Journal of Men's Studies, 9,* 41–57.

h. Volling, B. L., & Belsky, J. (1992). The contribution of mother-child and father-child relationships to the quality of sibling interaction: A longitudinal study. *Child Development, 63,* 1209–1222.

i Amato, P. R., & Rivera, F. (1999). Paternal involvement and children's behavior problems. *Journal of Marriage and the Family, 61,* 375–384; Rosenberg, J., & Wilcox, W. B. (2006). *The importance of fathers in the healthy development of children.* Washington, DC: U. S. Department of Health and Human Services, Administration for Children and Families, Administration on Children, Youth and Families, Children's Bureau, Office on Child Abuse and Neglect; Zimmerman, M. A., Salem, D. A., & Maton, K. I. (1995). Family structure and psychosocial correlates among urban African-American adolescent males. *Child Development, 66,* 1598–1613.

j. Dubowitz, H., Black, M. M., Cox, C. E., Kerr, M. A., Litrownik, A. J., Radhakrishna, A., et al. (2001). Father involvement and children's functioning at age 6 years: A multisite study. *Child Maltreatment, 6*(4), 300–309; Lamb, M. E. (Ed.). (1997). *The role of the father in child development* (3rd ed.). New York: John Wiley & Sons; Radin, N. (1972). Father-child interaction and the intellectual functioning of four-year-old boys. *Developmental Psychology, 6*(2), 353–361; Ricks, S. S. (1985). Father-infant interactions: A review of empirical research. *Family Relations, 34,* 505–511; Sutton-Smith, B., Rosenberg, B. G., & Landy, F. (1968). Father-absence effects in families of different sibling compositions. *Child Development, 39*(4), 1213–1221.

k. Browne, C. S., & Rife, J. C. (1991). Social, personality, and gender differences in at-risk and not-at-risk sixth-grade students. *Journal of Early Adolescence, 11*(4), 482–495; Harris, K. M., Furstenberg, F. F., Jr., & Marmer, J. K. (1998). Paternal involvement with adolescents in intact families: The influence of fathers over the life course. *Demography, 35*(2), 201–216; Nord, C. W., & West, J. (2001). *Fathers' and mothers' involvement in their children's schools by family type and resident status.* Washington, DC: National Center for Education Statistics, U.S. Department of Education; Rosenberg, J., & Wilcox, W. B. (2006). *The importance of fathers in the healthy development of children.* Washington, DC: U. S. Department of Health and Human Services, Administration for Children and Families, Administration on Children, Youth and Families, Children's Bureau, Office on Child Abuse and Neglect.

NOTES

CHAPTER 1

1. Bonner, J. T. (1988).The evolution of complexity by means of natural selection. Princeton, NJ: Princeton University Press.
2. Mesulam, M. M. (1998). From sensation to cognition. *Brain, 121,* 1013–1052.
3. Dunbar R. I. (1996). *Grooming, gossip, and the evolution of language.* Cambridge: Harvard University Press.
4. Simmons, L. W. (1945). *The role of the aged in primitive society.* New Haven: Shoe String Press.
5. Fischer, D. H. (1977). *Growing old in America.* New York: Oxford Press.
6. Shanas, E. (1968). *Old people in three industrial societies.* New York: Atherton Press.
7. Mahoney, D., & Restak, R. (1998). *The longevity strategy: How to live to 100 using the brain-body connection.* New York: John Wiley and Sons.
8. Bass, S. A., & Garo, F. G. (1996) The economic value of grandparent assistance. *Generations, 20*(1), 29–33.
9. LaDuke, W. (2005). *Recovering the sacred: The power of naming and claiming.* Cambridge, MA: South End Press.
10. Snowdon, D. (2001). *Aging with grace: What the nun study teaches us about leading longer, healthier, and more meaningful lives.* New York: Bantam Books.
11. Snowdon, D. (2001). *Aging with grace: What the nun study teaches us about leading longer, healthier, and more meaningful lives.* New York: Bantam Books.

CHAPTER 2

1. Cozolino, L. J. (2014). The neuroscience of human relationships: Attachment and the developing social brain (2nd ed.). New York: W. W. Norton & Company, Inc.
2. Stern, D. N. (1995). *The motherhood constellation.* New York: Basic Books.

3. Bugental, D. B., Martorell, G. A., & Barraza, V. (2003). The hormonal costs of subtle forms of infant maltreatment. *Hormones and Behavior, 43,* 237–244.

4. Cozolino, L. J. (2014). *The neuroscience of human relationships: Attachment and the developing social brain* (2ⁿᵈ ed.). New York: W. W. Norton & Company, Inc.

5. Barbas, H. (1995). Anatomic basis of cognitive-emotional interactions in the primate prefrontal cortex. *Neuroscience and Biobehavioral Reviews, 19,* 499–510; Porges, S. W. (2003). The polyvagal theory: Phylogenetic contributions to social behavior. *Physiology and Behavior, 79,* 503–513; Price, J. L. (1999). Prefrontal cortical networks related to visceral function and mood. *Annals of the New York Academy of Sciences, 877,* 383–396; Sullivan, R. M. & Gratton, A. (2002). Prefrontal cortical regulation of hypothalamic-pituitary-adrenal function in the rat and implications for psychopathology: Side matters. *Psychoneuroendocrinology, 27,* 99–114.

6. Allman, J., Hakeem, A., & Watson, K. (2002). Two phylogenetic specializations in the human brain. *Neuroscientist, 8,* 335–346; Nimchinsky, E. A., Gilissen, E., Allman, J. M., Perl, D. P., Erwin, J. M., & Hof, P. R. (1999). A neuronal morphologic type unique to humans and great apes. *Proceedings of the National Academy of Sciences, USA, 96,* 5268–5273.

7. Andersson, J. L. R., Lilja, A., Hartvif, P., Långström, B., Gordh, R., Handwerker, H., et al. (1997). Somatotopic organization along the central sulcus, for pain localization in humans, as revealed by psitron emission tomography. *Experimental Brain Research, 117,* 192–199; Bartels, A., & Zeki, S. (2000). The neural basis of romantic love. *NeuroReport, 11,* 3829–3834; Calder, A. J., Keane, J., Manly, T., Sprengelmeyer, R., Scott, S., Nimmo-Smith, S., et al. (2003). Facial expression recognition across the adult life span. *Neuropsychologia, 41,* 195–202; Phillips, M. L., Young, A. W., Senior, C., Brammer, M., Andrews, C., Calder, et al. (1997). A specific neural substrate for perceiving facial expressions of disgust. *Nature, 389,* 495–498.

8. Singer, T., Seymour, B., O'Doherty, J., Kaube, H., Dolan, R. J., & Frith, C. D. (2004). Empathy for pain involves the affective but not sensory components of pain. *Science, 303,* 1157–1162; Jackson, P. L., Meltzoff, A. N., & Decety, J. (2004). How do we perceive the pain of others? A window into the neural processes involved in empathy. *Neuroimage, 24,* 771–779.

9. Porges, S. W. (2003). The polyvagal theory: Phylogenetic contributions to social behavior. *Physiology and Behavior, 79,* 503–513.

10. Schultz, W., & Dickinson, A. (2000). Neuronal coding of prediction errors. *Annual Review of Neuroscience, 23,* 473–500.
11. Cumming, E., & Henry, W. E. (1961). *Growing old: The process of disengagement.* New York: Basic Books, Inc.

CHAPTER 3

1. Allen, J. S., Bruss, J., & Damasio, H. (2005). The aging brain: The cognitive reserve hypothesis and hominid evolution. *American Journal of Human Biology, 17,* 673–689; Charnov, E. L., & Berrigan, D. (1993). Why do female primates have such long lifespans and so few babies? Or life in the slow lane. *Evolutionary Anthropology, 1,* 191–194.
2. Kirkwood, T. B. L. (2002). Evolution of ageing. *Mechanisms of Ageing and Development, 123,* 737–745.
3. Lee, R. D. (2003). Rethinking the evolutionary theory of aging: Transfers, not births, shape senescence in social species. *Proceedings of the National Academy of Sciences, 100,* 9637–9642; Rogers, A. R. (1993). Why menopause? *Evolutionary Ecology, 7,* 406–420; Turke, P. W. (1997). Hypothesis: Menopause discourages infanticide and encourages continued investment by agnates. *Evolution and Human Behavior, 18,* 3–13.
4. Sear, R., Mace, R., & McGregor, I. A. (2000). Maternal grandmothers improve nutritional status and survival of children in rural Gambia. *Proceedings Biological Sciences, The Royal Society, 267,* 1641–1647.
5. Hawkes, K., O'Connell, J. F., & Jones, N. G. B. (1997). Hadza women's time allocation, offspring provisioning, and the evolution of long postmenopausal life spans. *Current Anthropology, 38,* 551–577; Lahdenperä, M., Lummaa, V., Helle, S., Tremblay, M., & Russell, A. F. (2004). Fitness benefits of prolonged post-reproductive lifespan in women. *Nature, 428,* 178–181; Pope, S. K., Whiteside, L., Brooks-Gunn, J., Kelleher, K. J., Rickert, V. I., Bradley, R. H., et al. (1993). Low-birth-weight infants born to adolescent mothers. Effects of coresidency with grandmother on child development. *JAMA, 269,* 1396–1400.
6. Jamison, C. S., Cornell, L. L., Jamison, P. L., & Nakazato, H. (2002). Are all grandmothers equal? A review and a preliminary test of the "grandmother hypothesis" in
7. Shanley, D. P., & Kirkwood, T. B. L. (2001). Evolution of the human menopause. *BioEssays, 23,* 282–287.
8. Szinovacz, M. E., & Davey, A. (2006). Effects of retirement and grandchild care on depressive symptoms. *International Journal of Aging and Human Development, 62,* 1–20; Thomas, J. L. (1986). Gender differences in satisfaction with grandparenting. *Psychology and Aging, 1,* 215–219.

9. Diamond, M. C., Johnson, R. E., & Ingham, C. (1971). Brain plasticity induced by environment and pregnancy. *International Journal of Neuroscience, 2*, 171–178.
10. Perls, T. T., Alpert, L., & Fretts, R. C. (1997). Middle-aged mothers live longer. *Nature, 389*, 133.
11. King, V., & Elder, G. H., Jr. (1997). The legacy of grandparenting: Childhood experiences with grandparents and current involvement with grandchildren. *Journal of Marriage and the Family, 59*, 848–859.
12. Robertson, J. F. (1977). Grandmotherhood: A study of role conceptions. *Journal of Marriage and Family, 39*(1), 165–174.
13. Baydar, N., & Brooks-Gunn, J. (1998). Profiles of grandmothers who help care for their grandchildren in the United States. *Family Relations, 47*, 385–393.
14. Bowers, B. F., & Myers, B. J. (1999). Grandmothers providing care for grandchildren: Consequences of various levels of caregiving. *Family Relations, 48*, 303–311
15. Burton, L. (1992). Black grandparents rearing children of drug-addicted parents: Stressors, outcomes, and social service needs. *Gerontologist, 32*, 744–751; Haglund, K. (2000). Parenting a second time around: An ethnography of African American grandmothers parenting grandchildren due to parental cocaine abuse. *Journal of Family Nursing, 6*, 120–135; Poindexter, C. C., & Linsk, N. L. (1999). "I'm just glad that I'm here": Stories of seven African-American HIV-affected grandmothers. *Journal of Gerontological Social Work, 32*, 63–81.
16. Kornhaber, A., & Woodward, K. L. (1981). *Grandparents/grandchildren: The vital connection.* Garden City, NY: Anchor Press/Doubleday.
17. Burton, L., & Devries, C. (1992). Challenges and rewards: African American grandparents as surrogate parents. *Generations, 16*, 51–54.
18. Jendrek, M. P. (1993). Grandparents who parent their grandchildren: Effects on lifestyle. *Journal of Marriage and the Family, 55*, 609–621.
19. Kivnick, H. Q. (1982). *The meaning of grandparenthood.* Ann Arbor, MI: UMI Research Press.
20. Waldrop, D. P., & Weber, J. A. (2001). From grandparent to caregiver: The stress and satisfaction of raising grandchildren. *Families in Society: The Journal of Contemporary Human Services, 5*, 461–472.
21. Coles, R. (1973). *The old ones of New Mexico.* Albuquerque: University of New Mexico Press.

CHAPTER 4

1. Wilson, E.O. (2012). *The Social Conquest of Earth*. New York, NY: W.W. Norton & Company Ltd.
2. Davidson, P. S. R., & Glisky, E. L. (2002). Neuropsychological correlates of recollection and familiarity in normal aging. *Cognitive, Affective, & Behavioral Neuroscience, 2*, 174–186.
3. Buonomano, D. V., & Merzenich, M. M. (1998). Cortical plasticity: From synapses to maps. *Annual Review of Neuroscience, 21*, 149–186; Trojan, S., & Pokorny, J. (1999). Theoretical aspects of neuroplasticity. *Physiological Research, 48*, 87–97.
4. Kempermann, G., Kuhn, H. G., & Gage, F. H. (1998). Experience-induced neurogenesis in the senescent dentate gyrus. *The Journal of Neuroscience, 18*(9), 3206–3212; Kolb, B., & Whishaw, I. Q. (1998). Brain plasticity and behavior. *Annual Review of Psychology, 49*, 43–64.
5. Diamond, M. C., Krech, D., & Rosenzweig, M. R. (1964). The effects of enriched environment on the histology of the rat cerebral cortex. *Journal of Comparative Neurology, 123*, 111–119; Guzowski, J. F., Setlow, B., Wagner, E. K., & McGaugh, J. L. (2001). Experience-dependent gene expression in the rat hippocampus after spatial learning: A comparison of the immediate-early genes Arc, c-fos, and zif268. *Journal of Neuroscience, 21*(14), 5089–5098; Ickes, B. R., Pham, T. M., Sanders, L. A., Albeck, D .S., Mohammed, A. H., & Grandholm, A. C. (2000). Long-term environmental enrichment leads to regional increases in neurotrophin levels in rat brains. *Experimental Neurology, 164*, 45–52.
6. Altman, J., Wallace, R. B., Anderson, W. J., & Das, G. D. (1968). Behaviorally induced changes in length of cerebrum in rats. *Developmental Psychobiology, 1*, 112–117; Kolb, B., & Gibb, R. (1991). Environmental enrichment and cortical injury: Behavioral and anatomical consequences of frontal cortex lesions. *Cerebral Cortex, 1*, 189–198; Schrott, L. M. (1997). Effect of training and environment on brain morphology and behavior. *Acta Paediatrica Scandanavia, 422*(Suppl.), 45–47; Schrott, L. M., Denenberg, V. H., Sherman, G. F., Waters, N. S., Rosen, G. D., & Galaburda, A. M. (1992). Environmental enrichment, neocortical ectopias, and behavior in the autoimmune NZB mouse. *Developmental Brain Research, 67*, 85–93; Schwartz, S. (1964). Effects of neonatal cortical lesions and early environmental factors on adult rat behavior. *Journal of Comparative Physiological Psychology, 57*, 72–77; Will, B. E., Rosenzweig, M. R., Bennett, E. B., Herbert, M., Morimoto,

H. (1977). Relatively brief environmental enrichment aids recovery of learning capacity and alters brain measures after postweaning brain lesions in rats. *Journal of Comparative Physiological Psychology, 91,* 33–50.

7. Anderson, S. W., Bechara, A., Damasio, H., Tranel, D., & Damasio, A.R. (2000). Acquisition of social knowledge is related to the prefrontal cortex. *Journal of Neurology, 247,* 72–73; Bartzokis, G., Cummings, J. L., Sultzer, D., Henderson, V. W., Nuechterlein, K. H., & Mintz, J. (2003). White matter structural integrity in healthy aging adults and patients with Alzheimer disease. *Archives of Neurology, 60,* 393–398; Braver, T. S., & Barch, D. M. (2002). A theory of cognitive control, aging cognition, and neuromodulation. *Neuroscience and Biobehavioral Reviews, 26,* 809–817; MacPherson, S. E., Phillips, L. H., & Della Salla, S. (2002). Age, executive function, and social decision making: A dorsolateral prefrontal theory of cognitive aging. *Psychology and Aging, 17,* 598–609; Rosen, A. C., Prull, M. W., O'Hara, R., Race, E. A., Desmond, J. E., Glover, G. H., et al. (2002). Variable effects of aging on frontal lobe contributions to memory. *Neuroreport, 13,* 2425–2428; Shan, Z. U., Liu, J. Z., Sahgal, V., Wang, B., & Yue, G. H. (2005). Selective atrophy of left hemisphere and frontal lobe of the brain in old men. *Journals of Gerontology: Biological Science, 60A,* 165–174; West, R. L. (1996). An application of prefrontal cortex function theory to cognitive aging. *Psychological Bulletin, 120,* 272–292.

8. MacPherson, S. E., Phillips, L. H., & Della Salla, S. (2002). Age, executive function, and social decision making: A dorsolateral prefrontal theory of cognitive aging. *Psychology and Aging, 17,* 598–609; Phillips, L. H., & Della Sala, S. (1998). Aging, intelligence, and anatomical segregation in the frontal lobes. *Learning and Individual Differences, 10,* 217–243.

9. Cornelius, S. W., & Caspi, A. (1987). Everyday problem solving in adulthood and old age. *Psychology and Aging, 2,* 144–153.

10. Leigland, L. A., Schulz, L. E., & Janowsky, J. S. (2004). Age related changes in emotional memory. *Neurobiology of Aging, 25,* 1117–1124.

11. Churchill, J. D., Stanis, J. J., Press, C., Kushelev, M., & Greenough, W. T. (2003). Is procedural memory relatively spared from age effects? *Neurobiology of Aging, 24,* 883–892; Rypma, B., & D'Esposito, M. (2000). Isolating the neural mechanisms of age-related changes in human working memory. *Nature Neuroscience, 3,* 509–515.

12. Haldane, J. B. S. (1941). *New Paths in Genetics.* London: George Allen & Unwin.

13. Rose, M. R. (1991). *Evolutionary biology of aging.* New York: Oxford University Press.

14. Williams, G. C. (1957). Pleiotropy, natural selection, and the evolution of senescence. *Evolution, 11,* 398–411.
15. Rose, M. R., & Mueller, L. D. (1998). Evolution of human lifespan: Past, future, and present. *American Journal of Human Biology, 10,* 409–420.
16. Ziuganov, V. V. (2005). A paradox of parasite prolonging the life of its host. Pearl mussel can disable the accelerated senescence program in salmon. *Biology Bulletin, 32,* 360–365.
17. Rose, M. R. (2005). *The long tomorrow: How advances in evolutionary biology can help us postpone aging.* New York: Oxford University Press.
18. Benes, F. M. (1989). Myelination of cortical-hippocampal relays during late adolescence. *Schizophrenia Bulletin, 15,* 585–593; Geuze, E., Vermetten, E., & Bremner, J. D. (2005). MR-based in vivo hippocampal volumetrics: 2. Findings in neuropsychiatric disorders. *Molecular Psychiatry, 10,* 160–184.
19. Sapolsky, R. M., Uno, H., Rebert, C. S., & Finch, C. E. (1990). Hippocampal damage associated with prolonged glucocorticoid exposure in primates. *Journal of Neuroscience, 10,* 2897–2902.
20. Kelly, A., Mullany, P. M., & Lynch, M. A. (2000). Protein synthesis in entorhinal cortex and long-term potentiation in dentate gyrus. *Hippocampus, 10,* 431–437; Pham, K., Nacher, J., Hof, P. R., & McEwen, B. (2003). Repeated restraint stress suppresses neurogenesis and induces biphasic PSA-NCAM expression in the adult rate dentate gyrus. *European Journal of Neuroscience, 17,* 879–886; Prickaerts, J., Koopmans, G., Blokland, A., & Scheepens, A. (2004). Learning and adult neurogenesis: Survival with or without proliferation? *Neurobiology of Learning and Memory, 81,* 1–11.
21. Lupien, S., de Leon, M., de Santi, S., Convit, A., Tarshish, C., Nair, N., et al. (1998). Cortisol levels during human aging predict hippocampal atrophy and memory deficits. *Nature Neuroscience, 1,* 69–73; West, M. J. (1993). Regionally specific loss of neurons in the aging human hippocampus. *Neurobiology of Aging, 14,* 287–293.
22. Bell, M. A., & Ball, M. J. (1981). Morphometric comparison of hippocampal microvasculature in ageing and demented people: Diameters and densities. *Acta Neuropathologica, 53,* 299–318; Black, J. E., Polinsky, M., & Greenough, W. T. (1989). Progressive failure of cerebral angiogenesis supporting neural plasticity in aging rats. *Neurobiology of Aging, 10,* 353–358; Keuker, J. I. H., Luiten, P. G. M., & Fuchs, E. (2000). Capillary changes in hippocampal CA1 and CA3 areas of the aging rhesus monkey. *Acta Neuropathologica, 100,* 665–672; Palmer, T. D., Willhoite, A. R., & Gage, F. H. (2000). Vascular niche for

adult hippocampal neurogenesis. *Journal of Comparative Neurology,* *425,* 479–494; Riddle, D. R., Sonntag, W. E., & Lichtenwalner, R. J. (2003). Microvascular plasticity in aging. *Ageing Research Reviews, 2,* 149–168.

23. DeCarli, C., Murphy, D. G. M., Gillette, J. A., Haxby, J. V., Teichberg, D., Schapiro, M. B., et al. (1994). Lack of age-related differences in temporal lobe volume of very healthy adults. *American Journal of Neuroradiology, 15,* 689–696.

24. Gazzaley, A. H., Weiland, N. G., McEwen, B. S., & Morrison, J. H. (1996). Differential regulation of NMDAR1 mRNA and protein by estradiol in the rat hippocampus. *Journal of Neuroscience, 16,* 6830–6838; Gooney, M., Messaoudi, E., Maher, F. O., Bramham, C. R., & Lynch, M. A. (2004). BDNF-induced LTP in dentate gyrus is impaired with age: Analysis of changes in cell signaling events. *Neurobiology of Aging, 25,* 1323–1331; Miller, D. B., & O'Callaghan, J. P, (2005). Aging, stress, and the hippocampus. *Ageing Research Reviews, 4,* 123–140; Sullivan, E. V., Marsh, L., & Pfefferbaum, A. (2005). Preservation of hippocampal volume throughout adulthood in healthy men and women. *Neurobiology of Aging, 26,* 1093–1098.

25. Esposito, G., Kirkby, B. S., Van Horn, J. D., Ellmore, T. M., & Berman, K. F. (1999). Context-dependent, neural system-specific neurophysiological concomitants of ageing: Mapping PET correlates during cognitive activation. *Brain, 122,* 963–979.

26. Beason-Held, L. L., Golski, S., Kraut, M. A., Esposito, G., & Resnick, S. M. (2005). Brain activation during encoding and recognition of verbal and figural information in older adults. *Neurobiology of Aging, 26,* 237–250; Logan, J. M., Sanders, A. L., Snyder, A. Z., Morris, J. C., & Buckner, R. L. (2002). Under-recruitment and nonselective recruitment: Dissociable neural mechanisms associated with aging. *Neuron, 33,* 827–840.

27. Li, K. Z. H., Lindenberger, U., Freund, A. M., & Baltes, P. B. (2001). Walking while memorizing: Age-related differences in compensatory behavior. *Psychological Science, 12,* 230–237; Nagahama, Y., Fukuyama, H., Yamauchi, H., Katsumi, Y., Magata, Y., Shibasaki, H., et al. (1997). Age-related changes in cerebral blood flow activation during a Card Sorting Test. *Experimental Brain Research, 114,* 571–577.

28. Heuninckx, S., Wenderoth, N., Debaere, F., Peeters, R., & Swinnen, S. P. (2005). Neural basis of aging: The penetration of cognition into action control. *Journal of Neuroscience, 25,* 6787–6796; Madden, D. J., Turkington, T. G., Provenzale, J. M., Denny, L. L., Hawk, T. C., Gottlob, L. R.,

et al. (1999). Adult age differences in the functional neuroanatomy of verbal recognition memory. *Human Brain Mapping, 7*, 115–135; Park, D. C., Welsh, R. C., Marshuetz, C., Gutchess, A. H., Mikels, J., Polk, T. A., et al. (2003). Working memory for complex scenes: Age differences in frontal and hippocampal activations. *Journal of Cognitive Neuroscience, 15*, 1122–1134.

29. Della-Maggiore, V., Sekuler, A. B., Grady, C. L., Bennett, P. J., Sekuler, R., & McIntosh, A. R. (2000). Corticolimbic interactions associated with performance on a short-term memory task are modified by age. *Journal of Neuroscience, 20*, 8410–8416.

30. Jacobs, B., Driscoll, L., & Schall, M. (1997). Life-span dendritic and spine changes in areas 10 and 18 of human cortex: A quantitative Golgi study. *Journal of Comparative Neurology, 386*, 661–680; Morrison, J. H., & Hof, P. R. (2003). Changes in cortical circuits during aging. *Clinical Neuroscience Research, 2*, 294–304.

31. Richards, M., & Deary, I. J. (2005). A life course approach to cognitive reserve: A model for cognitive aging and development? *Annals of Neurology, 58*, 617–622; Stern, Y., Alexander, G. E., Prohovnik, I., & Mayeux, R. (1992). Inverse relationship between educationand parieto-temporal perfusion deficit in Alzheimer's disease. *Annals of Neurology, 32*, 371–375.

32. Stern, Y., Habeck, C., Moeller, J., Scarmeas, N., Anderson, K. E., Hilton, H. J., et al. (2005). Brain networks associated with cognitive reserve in healthy young and old adults. *Cerebral Cortex, 15*, 394–402; Whalley, L. J., Deary, I. J., Appleton, C. L., & Starr, J. M. (2004). Cognitive reserve and the neurobiology of cognitive aging. *Ageing Research Reviews, 3*, 369–382.

33. Compton, D. M., Bachman, L. D., Brand, D., & Avet, T. L. (2000). Age-associated changes in cognitive function in highly educated adults: Emerging myths and realities. *International Journal of Geriatric Psychiatry, 15*, 75–85; Kessler, R. C., Berglund, P., Demler, O., Jin, R., Koretz, D., Merikangas, K. R., et al. (2003). The epidemiology of major depressive disorder: Results from the National Comorbidity Survey Replication (NCS-R). *Journal of American Medical Association, 289*, 3095–3105; Scarmeas, N., Zarahn, E., Anderson, K. E., Honig, L. S., Park, A., Hilton, J., et al. (2004). Cognitive reserve-mediated modulation of positron emission tomographic activations during memory tasks in Alzheimer disease. *Archives of Neurology, 61*, 73–78; Schmand, B., Smit, J. H., Geerlings, M. I., & Lindeboom, J. (1997). The effects of intelligence and education on the development of dementia: A test of the brain reserve

hypothesis. *Psychological Medicine, 27,* 1337–1344; Staff, R. T., Murray, A. D., Deary, I. J., & Whalley, L. J. (2004). What provides cerebral reserve? *Brain, 127,* 1191–1199; Stern, Y., Tang, M. X., Denaro, J., & Mayeux, R. (1995). Increased risk of mortality in Alzheimer's disease patients with more advanced educational and occupational attainment. *Annals of Neurology, 37,* 590–595.

34. Schaie, K. W., & Willis, S. L. (1986). Can decline in adult intellectual functioning be reversed? *Developmental Psychology, 22,* 223–232.

35. Riley, K. P., Snowdon, D. A., Desrosiers, M. F., & Markesbery, W. R. (2005). Early life linguistic ability, late life cognitive function, and neuropathology: Findings from the nun study. *Neurobiology of Aging, 26,* 341–347; Danner, D. D., Snowdon, D. A., & Friesen, W. V. (2001). Positive emotions in early life and longevity: Findings from the nun study. *Journal of Personality and Social Psychology, 80,* 804–813.

36. Ince, P. G. (2001). Pathological correlates of late-onset dementia in a multicentre, community-based population in England and Wales. *The Lancet, 357,* 169–175; Katzman, R., Aronson, M., Fuld, P., Kawas, C., Brown, T., Morgenstern, H., et al. (1989). Development of dementing illnessnes in an 80-year-old volunteer cohort. *Annals of Neurology, 25,* 317–324.

37. Alexander, G. E., Furey, M. L., Grady, C. L., Pietrini, P., Brady, D. R., Mentis, M. J., et al. (1997). Association of premorbid intellectual function with cerebral metabolism in Alzheimer's disease: Implications for the cognitive reserve hypothesis. *American Journal of Psychiatry, 154,* 165–172.

38. Ardila, A., Ostrosky-Solis, F., Rosselli, M., & Gomez, C. (2000). Age-related cognitive decline during normal aging: The complex effect of education. *Archives of Clinical Neuropsychology, 15,* 495–513; Le Carret, N., Lafont, S., Letenneur, L., Dartigues, J. F., Mayo, W., & Fabrigoule, C. (2003). The effect of education on cognitive performances and its implication for the constitution of the cognitive reserve. *Developmental Neuropsychology, 23,* 317–337.

39. Christensen, H., Henderson, A. S., Griffiths, K., & Levings, C. (1997). Does ageing inevitably lead to declines in cognitive performance? A longitudinal study of elite academics. *Personality and Individual Differences, 23,* 67–78.

40. Staff, R. T., Murray, A. D., Deary, I. J., & Whalley, L. J. (2004). What provides cerebral reserve? *Brain, 127,* 1191–1199.

41. Holloway, M. (2003). The mutable brain. *Scientific American, 289,* 78–85.

42. Jin, K., Sun, Y., Xie, L., Batteur, S., Mao, X. O., Smelick, C., et al. (2003). Neurogenesis and aging: FGF-2 and HB-EGF restore neurogenesis in hippocampus and subventricular zone of aged mice. *Aging Cell, 2*, 175–183; Johansson, B. B. (2004). Brain plasticity in health and disease. *Keio Journal of Medicine, 53*, 231–246; Kempermann, G., Gast, D., & Gage, F. H. (2002). Neuroplasticity in old age: Sustained fivefold induction of hippocampal neurogenesis by long-term environmental enrichment. *Annals of Neurology, 52*(2), 135–143.

CHAPTER 5

1. Bogin, B., & Smith, B. H. (1996). Evolution of the human life cycle. *American Journal of Human Biology, 8*, 703–716.
2. Canetti, L., Bachar, E., Galili-Weisstub, E., De-Nour, A. K., & Shalev, A. Y. (1997). Parental bonding and mental health in adolescence. *Adolescence, 32*, 381–394; Dahl, R. E. (2004). Adolescent brain development: A period of vulnerabilities and opportunities. *Annals of the New York Academy of Sciences, 1021*, 1–22.
3. Chambers, R. A., Taylor, J. R., & Potenza, M. N. (2003). Developmental neurocircuitry of motivation in adolescence: A critical period of addiction vulnerability. *American Journal of Psychiatry, 160*, 1041–1052; Rosenberg, D. R., & Lewis, D. A. (1995). Postnatal maturation of the dopaminergic innervation of monkey prefrontal and motor cortices: A tyrosine hydroxylase immunohistochemical analysis. *Journal of Comparative Neurology, 358*, 383–400; Spear, L. P. (2000). The adolescent brain and age-related behavioral manifestations. *Neuroscience and Biobehavioral Reviews, 24*, 417–463; Teicher, M. H., Andersen, S. L., & Hostetter, J. C. (1995). Evidence for dopamine receptor pruning between adolescence and adulthood in striatum but not nucleus accumbens. *Developmental Brain Research, 89*, 167–172.
4. Sowell, E. R., Thompson, P. M., Tessner, K. D., & Toga, A. W. (2001). Mapping continued brain growth and gray matter density reduction in dorsal frontal cortex: Inverse relationships during postadolescent brain maturation. *Journal of Neuroscience, 21*, 8819–8829.
5. Giedd, J. N. (2004). Structural magnetic resonance imaging of the adolescent brain. *Annals of the New York Academy of Sciences, 1021*, 77–85; Sowell, E. R., Trauner, D. A., Gamst, A., & Jernigan, T. L. (2002). Development of cortical and subcortical brain structures in childhood and adolescence: A structural MRI study. *Developmental Medicine & Child Neurology, 44*, 4–16.

6. Sowell, E. R., Thompson, P. M., Holmes, C. J., Jernigan, T. L., & Toga, A. W. (1999). In vivo evidence for post-adolescent brain maturation in frontal and striatal regions. *Nature Neuroscience, 2,* 859–861; Sowell, E. R., Thompson, P. M., Tessner, K. D., & Toga, A. W. (2001). Mapping continued brain growth and gray matter density reduction in dorsal frontal cortex: Inverse relationships during postadolescent brain maturation. *Journal of Neuroscience, 21,* 8819–8829.

7. Brown, T. T., Lugar, H. M., Coalson, R. S., Miezin, F. M., Petersen, S. E., & Schlaggar, B. L. (2005). Developmental changes in human cerebral functional organization for word generation. *Cerebral Cortex, 15,* 275–290; Schweinsburg, A. D., Nagel, B. J., Tapert S. F. (2005). fMRI reveals alteration of spatial working memory networks across adolescence. *Journal of the International Neuropsychological Society, 11,* 631–644.

8. Luna, B., & Sweeney, J. A. (2004). The emergence of collaborative brain function: fMRI studies of the development of response inhibition. *Annals of the New York Academy of Sciences, 1021,* 296–309; Pakkenberg, B., & Gundersen, H. J. G. (1997). Neocortical neuron number in humans: Effect of sex and age. *Journal of Comparative Neurology, 384,* 312–320.

9. Mesulam, M. M. (1987). Involutional and developmental implications of age-related neuronal changes: In search of an engram for wisdom. *Neurobiology of Aging, 8,* 581–583; Petrella, J. R., Townsend, B. A., Jha, A. P., Ziajko, L. A., Slavin, M. J., Lustig, C., et al. (2005). Increasing memory load modulates regional brain activity in older adults as measured by fMRI. *Journal of Neuropsychiatry Clinical Neuroscience, 17,* 75–84.

10. Rose, M. R. (1991). *Evolutionary biology of aging.* New York: Oxford University Press.

11. Stern, Y., Habeck, C., Moeller, J., Scarmeas, N., Anderson, K. E., Hilton, H. J., et al. (2005). Brain networks associated with cognitive reserve in healthy young and old adults. *Cerebral Cortex, 15,* 394–402.

12. Anokhin, A. P., Birbaumer, N., Lutzenberger, W., Nikolaev, A., & Vogel, F. (1996). Age increases brain complexity. *Electroencephalography and clinical neurophysiology, 99,* 63–68.

13. Grieve, S. M., Clark, C. R., Williams, L. M., Peduto, A. J., & Gordon, E. (2005). Preservation of limbic and paralimbic structures in aging. *Human Brain Mapping, 25,* 391–401; Whalley, L. J. (2001). *The aging brain.* New York: Columbia University Press.

14. Giannakopoulos, P., Hof, P. R., Michel, J.-P., Guimon, J., & Bouras, C. (1997). Cerebral cortex pathology in aging and Alzheimer's disease: A quantitative survey of large hospital-based geriatric and psy-

chiatric cohorts. *Brain Research Reviews*, 25, 217–245; Head, D., Snyder, A. Z., Girton, L. E., Morris, J. C., & Buckner, R. L. (2005). Frontal-hippocampal double dissociation between normal aging and Alzheimer's disease. *Cerebral Cortex*, 15, 732–739.

15. Happé, F. G. E., Winner, E., & Brownell, H. (1998). The getting of wisdom: Theory of mind in old age. *Developmental Psychology*, 34, 358–362.

16. United Nations Department of Economic and Social Affairs Population Division. (1998). *World Population Prospects* (1998 Revision). New York, NY: Author.

17. Mueller, E. A., Moore, M. M., Kerr, D. C. R., Sexton, G., Camicioli, R. M., Howieson, D. B., et al. (1998). Brain volume preserved in healthy elderly through the eleventh decade. *Neurology*, 51, 1555–1562.

18. Perls, T. T. (2004). The oldest old. *Scientific American*, 272, *The Science of Staying Young* [Special Issue], 6–11.

19. Erraji-Benchekroun, L., Underwood, M. D., Arango, V., Galfavy, H., Pavlidis, P., Smyrniotopoulous, P., et al. (2005). Molecular aging in human prefrontal cortex is selective and continuous throughout adult life. *Biological Psychiatry*, 57, 549–558.

20. Baptista, L. F., & Petrinovich, L. (1986). Song development in the white-crowned sparrow: Social factors and sex differences. *Animal Behavior*, 34, 1359–1371.

21. Eales, L. A. (1985). Song learning in zebra finches: Some effects of song model availability on what is learnt and when. *Animal Behavior*, 37, 507–508.

CHAPTER 6

1. Rattenborg, N. C., Amlaner, C. J., & Lima, S. L. (2000). Behavioral, neurophysiological and evolutionary perspectives on unihemispheric sleep. *Neuroscience and Biobehavioral Reviews*, 24, 817–842.

2. Ringo, J. L., Dory, R. W., Demeter, S., & Simard, P. Y. (1994). Time is of the essence: A conjecture that hemispheric specialization arises from interhemispheric conduction delay. *Cerebral Cortex*, 4, 331–343.

3. Berrebi, A. S., Fitch, R. H., Ralphe, D. L., Denenberg, J. O., Friedrich, V. L., Jr., & Denenberg, V. H. (1988). Corpus callosum: Region-specific effects of sex, early experience and age. *Brain Research*, 438, 216–224.

4. Anderson, B., & Rutledge, V. (1996). Age and hemisphere effects on dendritic structure. *Brain*, 119, 1983–1990.

5. Liederman, J., & Meehan, P. (1986). When is between-hemisphere division of labor advantageous? *Neuropsychologia*, 24, 863–874.

6. Cabeza, R., Anderson, N. D., Houle, S., Mangels, J. A., & Nyberg, L. (2000). Age-related differences in neural activity during item and temporal-order memory retrieval: A positron emission tomography study. *Journal of Cognitive Neuroscience, 12*, 197–206.

7. Levine, B. (2004). Autobiographical memory and the self in time: Brain lesion effects, functional neuroanatomy, and lifespan development. *Brain and Cognition, 55*, 54–68.

8. Anokhin, A. P., Birbaumer, N., Lutzenberger, W., Nikolaev, A., & Vogel, F. (1996). Age increases brain complexity. *Electroencephalography and clinical neurophysiology, 99*, 63–68; Tessitore, A., Hariri, A. R., Fera, F., Smith, W. G., Das, S., Weinberger, D. R. et al. (2005). Functional changes in the activity of brain regions underlying emotion processing in the elderly. *Psychiatry Research: Neuroimaging, 139*, 9–18.

9. Cabeza, R., Anderson, N. D., Locantore, J. K., & McIntosh, A. (2002). Aging gracefully: Compensatory brain activity in high-performing older adults. *NeuroImage, 17*, 1394–1402.

10. Vaillant, G. E. (2002). *Aging well.* New York: Little, Brown and Company.

11. Arnold, A. P. (2004). Sex chromosomes and brain gender. *Neuroscience, 5*, 1–8.

12. Zelditch, M. (1955). Role differentiation in the nuclear family. In T. Parsons & R. F. Bales (Eds.), *Family, socialization and interaction process* (pp. 307–352). Glencoe, IL: Free Press.

13. Carne, R. P., Vogrin, S., Litewka, L., & Cook, M. J. (2006). Cerebral cortex: An MRI-based study of volume and variance with age and sex. *Journal of Clinical Neuroscience, 13*, 60–72; Cowell, P. E., Turetsky, B. I., Gur, R. C., Grossman, R. I., Shtasel, D. L., & Gur, R. E. (1994). Sex differences in aging of the human frontal and temporal lobes. *Journal of Neuroscience, 14*, 4748–4755; Gur, R. C., Mozley, P. D., Resnick, S. M., Gottlieb, G. L., Kohn, M., Zimmerman, R., et al. (1991). Gender differences in age effect on brain atrophy measured by magnetic resonance imaging. *Proceedings of the National Academy of Sciences, USA, 88*, 2845–2849; Shan, Z. U., Liu, J. Z., Sahgal, V., Wang, B., & Yue, G. H. (2005). Selective atrophy of left hemisphere and frontal lobe of the brain in old men. *Journals of Gerontology: Biological Science, 60A*, 165–174; Xu, J., Kobayashi, S., Yamaguchi, S., Iijima, K., Okada, K., & Yamashita, K. (2000). Gender effects on age-related changes in brain structure. *American Journal of Neuroradiology, 21*, 112–118.

14. Witelson, S. F., Beresh, H., & Kigar, D. L. (2006). Intelligence and brain size in 100 postmortem brains: Sex, lateralization and age factors. *Brain, 129*, 386–398.

15. Frings, L., Wagner, K., Unterrainer, J., Spreer, J., Halsband, U., & Schulze-Bonhage, A. (2006). Gender-related differences in lateralization of hippocampal activation and cognitive strategy. *Brain Imaging, 17,* 417–421.

16. Bell, E. C., Willson, M. C., Wilman, A. H., Dave, S., & Silverstone, P. H. (2006). Males and females differ in brain activation during cognitive tasks. *NeuroImage, 30,* 529–538; Johnson, E. S., & Meade, A. C. (1987). Developmental patterns of spatial ability: An early sex difference. *Child Development, 58,* 725–740; Kawachi, T., Ishii, K., Sakamoto, S., Matsui, M., Mori, T., & Sasaki, M. (2002). Gender differences in cerebral glucose metabolism: A PET study. *Journal of the Neurological Sciences, 199,* 79–83; Piefke, M., Weiss, P. H., Markowitsch, H. J., & Fink, G. R. (2005). Gender differences in functional neuroanatomy of emotional episodic autobiographical memory. *Human Brain Mapping, 24,* 313–324; Riello, R., Sabattoli, F., Beltramello, A., Bonetti, M., Bono, G., Falini, A., et al. (2005). Brain volumes in healthy adults aged 40 years and over: A voxel-based morphometry study. *Aging and Clinical Experimental Research, 17,* 329–336; Schlaepfer, T. E., Harris, G. J., Tien, A. Y., Peng, L., Lee, S., & Pearlson, G. D. (1995). Structural differences in the cerebral cortex of healthy female and male subjects: An MRI study. *Psychiatry Research – Neuroimaging, 61,* 129–135; Vederhus, L., & Krekling, S. (1996). Sex differences in visual spatial ability in 9-year-old children. *Intelligence, 23,* 33–43.

17. Allen, L. S., & Gorski, R. A. (1991). Sexual dimorphism of the anterior commissure and massa intermedia of the human brain. *Journal of Comparative Neurology, 312,* 97–104; Sullivan, E. V., Rosenbloom, M. J., Desmond, J. E., & Pfefferbaum, A. (2001). Sex differences in corpus callosum size: Relationship to age and intracranial size. *Neurobiology of Aging, 22,* 603–611.

18. Cowell, P. E., Allen, L. S., Zalatimo, N. S., & Denenberg, V. H. (1992). A developmental study of sex and age interactions in the human corpus callosum. *Developmental Brain Research, 66,* 187–192.

19. Sullivan, E. V., Rosenbloom, M. J., Desmond, J. E., & Pfefferbaum, A. (2001). Sex differences in corpus callosum size: Relationship to age and intracranial size. *Neurobiology of Aging, 22,* 603–611.

20. Eals, M., & Silverman, I. (1994). The hunter-gatherer theory of spatial sex differences: Proximate factors mediating the female advantage in recall of object arrays. *Ethology and Sociobiology, 15,* 95–105; Kimura, D. (1992). Sex differences in the brain. *Scientific American, 267,* 118–125; McBurney, D. H., Gaulin, S. J. C., Devineni, T., & Adams, C. (1997).

Superior spatial memory of women: Stronger evidence for the gathering hypothesis. *Evolution and Human Behavior, 18,* 165–174; Ward, S. L., Newcombe, N., & Overton, W. F. (1986). Turn left at the church, or three miles north: A study of direction giving and sex differences. *Environment and Behavior, 18,* 192–213.

21. Taylor, S. E., Klein, L. C., Lewis, B. P., Gruenewald, T. L., Gurung, R. A. R., & Updegraff, J. A. (2000). Biobehavioral response to stress in females: Tend-and-befriend, not fight-or-flight. *Psychological Review, 107,* 411–429.

22. Kamil, A. C. (2004). Sociality and the evolution of intelligence. *Trends in Cognitive Sciences, 8,* 195–197.

23. Cherrier, M. M., Matsumoto, A. M., Amory, J. K., Ahmed, S., Bremner, W., Peskind, E. R., et al. (2005). The role of aromatization in testosterone supplementation: Effects on cognition in older men. *Neurology, 64,* 290–296.

24. Shugrue, P. J., & Merchenthaler, I. (2000). Estrogen is more than just a "sex hormone": Novel sites for estrogen action in the hippocampus and cerebral cortex. *Frontiers in Neuroendocrinology, 21,* 95–101.

25. Hammond, J., Le, Q., Goodyer, C., Gelfand, M., Trifiro, M., & LeBlanc, A. (2001). Testosterone-mediated neuroprotection through the androgen receptor in human primary neurons. *Journal of Neurochemistry, 77,* 1319–1326; Takao, T., Flint, N., Lee, L., Ying, X., Merrill, J., & Chandross, K. J. (2004). 17beta-estradiol protects oligodendrocytes from cytotoxicity induced cell death. *Journal of Neurochemistry, 89,* 660–673.

26. Adams, M. M., Shah, R. A., Janssen, W. G. M., & Morrison, J. H. (2001). Different modes of hippocampal plasticity in response to estrogen in young and aged female rats. *Proceedings of the National Academy of Sciences, USA, 98,* 8071–8076; Gazzaley, A. H., Weiland, N. G., McEwen, B. S., & Morrison, J. H. (1996). Differential regulation of NMDAR1 mRNA and protein by estradiol in the rat hippocampus. *Journal of Neuroscience, 16,* 6830–6838. Behl, C., Widmann, M., Trapp, T., & Holsboer, F. (1995). 17-beta estradiol protects neurons from oxidative stress-induced cell death in vitro. *Biochemical and Biophysical Research Communications, 216,* 473–482; Behl, C., Skutella, T., Lezoualc'h, F., Post, A., Widmann, M., Newton, C. J., et al. (1997). Neuroprotection against oxidative stress by estrogens: Structure-activity relationship. *Molecular Pharmacology, 51,* 535–541; Takao, T., Flint, N., Lee, L., Ying, X., Merrill, J., & Chandross, K. J. (2004). 17beta-estradiol protects oligodendrocytes from cytotoxicity induced cell death. *Journal of Neurochemistry, 89,* 660–673.

27. Register, T. C., Shivley, C. A., & Lewis, C. E. (1998). Expression of estrogen receptor alpha and beta transcripts in female monkey hippocampus and hypothalamus. *Brain Research, 788*, 320–322.

28. Hampson, E. (1990). Estrogen-related variations in human spatial and articulatory-motor skills. *Psychoneuroendocrinology, 15*, 97–111; Hampson, E., & Kimura, D. (1988). Reciprocal effects of hormonal fluctuations on human motor and perceptual-spatial skills. *Behavioral Neuroscience, 102*, 456–459.

29. Aleman, A., Bronk, E., Kessels, R. P. C., Koppeschaar, H. P. F., & van Honk, J. (2004). A single administration of testosterone improves visuospatial ability in young women. *Psychoneuroendocrinology, 29*, 612–617; Wang, C., Swerdloff, R. S., Iranmanesh, A., Dobs, A., Snyder, P. J., Cunningham, G., et al. (2000). Transdermal testosterone gel improves sexual function, mood, muscle strength, and body composition paramenters in hypogonadal men. *Journal of Clinical Endocrinology and Metabolism, 85*, 2839–2853.

30. Moffat, S. D., Zonderman, A. B., Metter, E. J., Blackman, M. R., Harman, S. M., & Resnick, S. M. (2002). Longitudinal assessment of serum free testosterone concentration predicts memory performance and cognitive status in elderly men. *Journal of Clinical Endocrinology & Metabolism, 87*, 5001–5007; Moffat, S. D., Zonderman, A. B., Metter, E. J., Kawas, C., Blackman, M. R., Harman, S. M., et al. (2004). Free testosterone and risk for Alzheimer disease in older men. *Neurology, 62*, 188–193; Raber, J., Bongers, G., LeFevour, A., Buttini, M., & Mucke, L. (2002). Androgens protect against apolipoprotein E4-induced cognitive deficits. *Journal of Neuroscience, 22*, 5204–5209.

CHAPTER 7

1. Twain, M. (1965). *The adventures of Huckleberry Finn*. New York: Bantam Books.

2. Sternberg, R. J. (Ed.). (1990). *Wisdom: Its nature, origins, and development*. New York: Cambridge University Press.

3. Takahashi, M., & Bordia, P. (2000). The concept of wisdom: A cross-cultural comparison. *International Journal of Psychology, 35*, 1–9.

4. Ardelt, M. (2004). Where can wisdom be found? A reply to the commentaries by Baltes and Kunzmann, Sternberg, and Achenbaum. *Human Development, 47*, 304–307.

5. Siegel, D. J. (2017). *Mind: A journey to the heart of being human*. New York: W.W. Norton & Company; Takahashi, M., & Overton, W. F.

(2002). Wisdom: A culturally inclusive developmental perspective. *International Journal of Behavioral Development, 26*, 269–277.

6. Staudinger, U. M., & Baltes, P. B. (1996). Interactive minds: A facilitative setting for wisdom-related performance? *Journal of Personality and Social Psychology, 71*, 746–762.

7. Paulhus, D. L., Wehr, P., Harms, P. D., & Strasser, D. I. (2002). Use of exemplar surveys to reveal implicit types of intelligence. *Personality and Social Psychology Bulletin, 28*, 1051–1062.

8. Staudinger, U. M. (1999). Older and wiser? Integrating results on the relationship between age and wisdom-related performance. *International Journal of Behavioral Development, 23*, 641–664.

9. Baltes, P. B., Staudinger, U. M., Maercker, A., & Smith, J. (1995). People nominated as wise: A comparative study of wisdom-related knowledge. *Psychology and Aging, 10*, 155–166.

10. Staudinger, U. M., Maciel, A. G., Smith, J., & Baltes, P. B. (1998). What predicts wisdom-related performance? A first look at personality, intelligence, and facilitative experiential contexts. *European Journal of Personality, 12*, 1–17.

11. Holliday, S. G., & Chandler, M. J. (1986). *Wisdom: Explorations in adult competence.* New York: Karger.

12. Pliske, R. M., & Mutter, S. A. (1996). Age differences in the accuracy of confidence judgments. *Experimental Aging Research, 22*, 199–216; Staudinger, U. M., Maciel, A. G., Smith, J., & Baltes, P. B. (1998). What predicts wisdom-related performance? A first look at personality, intelligence, and facilitative experiential contexts. *European Journal of Personality, 12*, 1–17.

13. McAdams, D. P., St. Aubin, E. D., & Logan, R. L. (1993). Generativity among young, midlife, and older adults. *Psychology and Aging, 8*, 221–230;

14. Vaillant, G. E. (2002). *Aging well.* New York: Little, Brown and Company.

15. Pasupathi, M., & Staudinger, U. M. (2001). Do advanced moral reasoners also show wisdom? Linking moral reasoning and wisdom-rleated knowledge and judgment. *International Journal of Behavioral Development, 25*(5), 401–415.

16. Danner, D. D., Snowdon, D. A., & Friesen, W. V. (2001). Positive emotions in early life and longevity: Findings from the nun study. *Journal of Personality and Social Psychology, 80*, 804–813.

17. Ardelt, M. (1997). Wisdom and life satisfaction in old age. *Journal of Gerontology: Psychological Sciences, 52B*, P15–P27; Ardelt, M. (2000).

Antecedents and effects of wisdom in old age: A longitudinal perspective on aging well. *Research on Aging, 22,* 360–394.

18. Baltes, M., & Lang, F. (1997). Everyday functioning and successful aging: The impact of resources. *Psychology and Aging, 12,* 433–443.

CHAPTER 8

1. Davis, M. (2002). Role of NMDA receptors and MAP kinase in the amygdala in extinction of fear: Clinical implications for exposure therapy. *European Journal of Neuroscience, 16,* 395–398.
2. Ballmaier, M., Toga, A. W., Blanton, R. E., Sowell, E. R., Lavretsky, H., Peterson, J., et al. (2004). Anterior cingulate, gyrus rectus, and orbitofrontal abnormalities in elderly depressed patients: An MRI-based parcellation of the prefrontal cortex. *American Journal of Psychiatry, 161,* 99–108; Lai, T.-J., Payne, M. E., Byrum, C. E., Steffens, D. C., & Krishnan, K. R. R. (2000). Reduction of orbital frontal cortex volume in geriatric depression. *Biological Psychiatry, 48,* 971–975; Taylor, W. D., Steffens, D. C., McQuoid, D. R., Payne, M. E., Lee, S.-H., Lai, T.-J., et al. (2003). Smaller orbital frontal cortex volumes associated with functional disability in depressed elders. *Biological Psychiatry, 53,* 144–149.
3. O'Doherty, J. Kringelbach, M. L., Rolls, E. T., Hornak, J., & Andrews, C. (2001). Abstract reward and punishment representations in the human orbitofrontal cortex. *Nature Neuroscience, 4,* 95–102.
4. Hendler, T., Rotshtein, P., Yeshurun, Y., Weizmann, T., Kahn, I. Ben-Bashat, D., et al. (2003). Sensing the invisible: Differential sensitivity of visual cortex and amygdala to traumatic context. *Neuroimage, 19,* 587–600; Morris, J. S., Öhman, A., & Dolan, R. J. (1998). Conscious and unconscious emotional learning in the human amygdala. *Nature, 393,* 467–470; Morris, J. S., Öhman, A., & Dolan, R. J. (1999). A subcortical pathway to the right amygdala: Mediating "unseen" fear. *Proceedings of the National Academy of Sciences, USA, 96,* 1680–1685.
5. Gur, R. C., Schroeder, L., Turner, T., McGrath, C., Chan, R. M., Turetsky, B. I., et al. (2002). Brain activation during facial emotion processing. *NeuroImage, 16,* 651–662; Rule, R. R., Shimamura, A. P., & Knight, R. T. (2002). Orbitofrontal cortex and dynamic filtering of emotional stimuli. *Cognitive, Affective, & Behavioral Neuroscience, 2,* 264–270; Schaefer, S. M. (2002). Modulation of amygdalar activity by the conscious regulation of negative emotion. *Journal of Cognitive Neuroscience, 14,* 913–921; Simpson, J. R., Drevets, W. C., Snyder, A. Z., Gusnard, D. A., & Raichle, M. E. (2001). Emotion-induced changes in human medial prefrontal cortex: II. During anticipatory anxiety. *Pro-*

ceedings of the National Academy of Sciences, 98, 688–693; Simpson, J. R., Snyder, A. Z., Gusnard, D. A., & Raichle, M. E. (2001). Emotional-induced changes in human medial prefrontal cortex: I. During cognitive task performance. Proceedings of the National Academy of Sciences, USA, 98, 683–687.

6. Drevets, W. C., & Raichle, M. E. (1998). Reciprocal Suppression of regional cerebral blood during emotional versus higher cognitive processes: Implications for interactions between emotion and cognition. Cognition and Emotion, 12, 353–385; Kim, H., Somerville, L. H., Johnstone, T., Alexander, A. L., & Whalen, P. J. (2003). Inverse amygdala and medial prefrontal cortex responses to surprised faces. NeuroReport, 14, 2317–2322; Nomura, M., Ohira, H., Haneda, K., Iidaka, T., Sadato, N., Okada, T., et al. (2004). Functional association of the amygdala and ventral prefrontal cortex during cognitive evaluation of facial expressions primed by masked angry faces: An event-related fMRI study. NeuroImage, 21, 352–363; Shin, L. M., Wright, C. I., & Cannistraro, P. A. (2005). A functional magnetic resonance imaging study of amygdala and medial prefrontal cortex responses to overtly presented fearful faces in posttraumatic stress disorder. Archives of General Psychiatry, 62, 273–281; Yamasaki, H., LaBar, K. S., & McCarthy, G. (2002). Dissociable prefrontal brain systems for attention and emotion. Proceedings of the National Academy of Sciences, USA, 99, 11447–11451.

7. Nader, K. (2003). Memory traces unbound. Trends in Neurosciences, 26, 65–72.

8. Rainnie, D. G., Bergeron, R., Sajdyk, T. J., Patil, M., Gehlert, D. R., & Shekhar, A. (2004). Corticotrophin releasing factor-induced synaptic plasticity in the amygdala translates stress into emotional disorders. Journal of Neuroscience, 24, 3471–3479; Vyas, A., Mitra, R., Shankaranarayana Rao, B. S., & Chattarji, S. (2002). Chronic stress induces contrasting patterns of dendritic remodeling in hippocampal and amygdaloid neurons. Journal of Neuroscience, 22, 6810–6818; Vyas, A., & Chattarji, S. (2004). Modulation of different states of anxiety-like behavior by chronic stress. Behavioral Neuroscience, 118, 1450–1454.

9. Allman, J., McLaughlin, T., & Hakeem, A. (1993). Brain structures and life-span in primate species. Proceedings of the National Academy of Sciences, 90, 3359–3563.

10. De Bellis, M. D., Casey, B. J., Dahl, R. E., Birmaher, B., Williamson, D. E., Thomas, K. M., et al. (2000). A pilot study of amygdala volumes in pediatric generalized anxiety disorder. Biological Psychiatry, 48, 51–57.

11. Ito, T. A., Larsen, J. T., Smith, N. K., & Cacioppo, J. T. (2002). Negative information weighs more heavily on the brain: The negativity bias in evaluative categorizations. In J. T. Cacioppo, G. C. Berntson, R. Adolphs, C. S. Carter, R. J. Davidson, & M. K. McClintock, et al. (Eds.), Foundations in social neuroscience (pp.575–597). Massachusetts: MIT Press.

12. McEchron, M. D., Cheng, A. Y., & Gilmartin, M. R. (2004). Trace fear conditioning is reduced in the aging rat. Neurobiology of Learning and Memory, 82, 71–76; Torras-Garcia, M., Costa-Miserachs, D., Coll-Andreu, M., & Portell-Cortes, I. (2005). Decreased anxiety levels related to aging. Experimental Brain Research, 164, 177–184.

13. Tessitore, A., Hariri, A. R., Fera, F., Smith, W. G., Das, S., Weinberger, D. R. et al. (2005). Functional changes in the activity of brain regions underlying emotion processing in the elderly. Psychiatry Research: Neuroimaging, 139, 9–18.

14. Wright, C. I., Wedig, M. M., Williams, D., Rauch, S. L., & Albert, M. S. (2006). Novel fearful faces activate the amygdala in healthy young and elderly adults. Neurobiology of Aging, 27, 361–374.

15. Tsai, J. L., Levenson, R. W., & Carstensen, L. L. (2000). Autonomic, subjective, and expressive responses to emotional films in older and younger Chinese Americans and European Americans. Psychology and Aging, 15, 684–693.

16. De Martino, B., Kumaran, D., Seymour, B., & Dola, R. J. (2006). Frames, biases, and rational decision-making in the human brain. Science, 313(5787), 684–687.

17. Blanchard-Fields, F. (1986). Reasoning on social dilemmas varying in emotional saliency: An adult developmental perspective. Psychology and Aging, 1, 325–333; Blanchard-Fields, F., & Irion, J. C. (2001). Coping strategies from the perspective of two developmental markers: Age and social reasoning. Journal of Genetic Psychology, 149, 141–151.

18. Carstensen, L. L., Pasupathi, M., Mayr, U., & Nesselroade, J. R. (2000). Emotional experience in everyday life across the adult life span. Journal of Personality and Social Psychology, 79, 644–655.

19. Gross, J. J., Carstensen, L. L., Pasupathi, M., Tsai, J., Skorpen, C. G., & Hsu, A. Y. C. (1997). Emotion and aging: Experience, expression, and control. Psychology and Aging, 12, 590–599.

20. Mroczek, D. K., & Kolarz, C. M. (1998). The effect of age on positive and negative affect: A developmental perspective on happiness. Journal of Personality and Social Psychology, 75, 1333–1349.

21. Charles, S. T., Mather, M., & Carstensen, L. L. (2003). Aging and emo-

tional memory: The forgettable nature of negative images for older adults. *Journal of Experimental Psychology, 132,* 310–324; Pasupathi, M., & Carstensen, L. L. (2003). Age and emotional experience during mutual reminiscing. *Psychology and Aging, 18,* 430–442.

22. Iidaka, T., Okada, T., Murata, T., Omori, M., Kosaka, H., Sadato, N., et al. (2002). Age-related differences in the medial temporal lobe responses to emotional faces as revealed by fMRI. *Hippocampus, 12,* 352–362; Mather, M., & Carstensen, L. L. (2003). Aging and attentional biases for emotional faces. *Psychological Science, 14,* 409–415.

23. Mather, M., Canli, T., English, T., Whitfield, S., Wais, P., Ochsner, K., et al. (2004). Amygdala responses to emotionally valenced stimuli in older and younger adults. *Psychological Science, 15,* 259–263.

24. Gunning-Dixon, F. M., Gur, R. C., Perkins, A. C., Schroeder, L., Turner, T., Turetsky, B. I., et al. (2003). Age-related differences in brain activation during emotional face processing. *Neurobiology of Aging, 24,* 285–295.

25. LaBar, K. S., & Cabeza, R. (2006). Cognitive neuroscience of emotional memory. *Nature Reviews. Neuroscience, 7*(1), 54–64; Leigland, L. A., Schulz, L. E., & Janowsky, J. S. (2004). Age related changes in emotional memory. *Neurobiology of Aging, 25,* 1117–1124; Cahill, L., & McGaugh, J. L. (1996). Modulation of memory storage. *Current Opinion in Neurobiology, 6,* 237–242; Tessitore, A., Hariri, A. R., Fera, F., Smith, W. G., Das, S., Weinberger, D. R. et al. (2005). Functional changes in the activity of brain regions underlying emotion processing in the elderly. *Psychiatry Research: Neuroimaging, 139,* 9–18.

26. Mather, M., Canli, T., English, T., Whitfield, S., Wais, P., Ochsner, K., et al. (2004). Amygdala responses to emotionally valenced stimuli in older and younger adults. *Psychological Science, 15,* 259–263;

27. Kennedy, Q., Mather, M., & Carstensen, L. L. (2004). The role of motivation in the age-related positivity effect in autobiographical memory. *Psychological Science, 15,* 208–214; Leigland, L. A., Schulz, L. E., & Janowsky, J. S. (2004). Age related changes in emotional memory. *Neurobiology of Aging, 25,* 1117–1124.

28. Taylor, S. E., Kemeny, M. E., Reed, G. M., Bower, J. E., & Gruenewald, T. L. (2000). Psychological resources, positive illusions, and health. *American Psychologist, 55*(1), 99–109.

29. Maruta, T., Colligan, R. C., Malinchoc, M. & Offord, K. P. (2002). Optimism-pessimism assessed in the 1960s and self-reported health status 30 years later. *Mayo Clinic Proceedings, 77,* 748–753; Peterson, C., Seligman, M. E. P., & Vaillant, G. E. (1988). Pessimistic explanatory

style is a risk factor for physical illness: A thirty-five-year longitudinal study. *Journal of Personality and Social Psychology, 55,* 23–27.

30. Allison, P., Guichard, C., Fung, K., & Gilain, L. (2003). Dispositional optimism predicts survival status 1 year after diagnosis in head and neck cancer patients. *Journal of Clinical Oncology, 21*(3), 543–8; Fredrickson, B. L. & Levenson, R. W. (1998). Positive emotions speed recovery from the cardiovascular sequelae of negative emotions. *Cognition and Emotion, 12*(2), 191–220; Scheier, M. F., Matthews, K. A., Owens, J. F., Schulz, R., Bridges, M. W., Magovern, G. J. et al. (1999). Optimism and rehospitalization after coronary artery bypass graft surgery. *Archives of Internal Medicine, 159,* 829–835.

31. Carver, C. S., Pozo, C., Harris, S. D., Noriega, V., Scheier, M. F., Robinson, D. S. et al. (1993). How coping mediates the effect of optimism on distress: A study of women with early stage breast cancer. *Journal of Personality and Social Psychology, 65*(2), 375–390.

32. Maroto, J. J., Pbert, L. A., & Shepperd, J. A. (1996). Dispositional optimism as a predictor of health changes among cardiac patients. *Journal of Research in Personality, 30,* 517–534; Scheier, M. F., Matthews, K. A., Owens, J. F., Schulz, R., Bridges, M. W., Magovern, G. J. et al. (1999). Optimism and rehospitalization after coronary artery bypass graft surgery. *Archives of Internal Medicine, 159,* 829–835.

33. Ironson, G., Balbin, E., Stuetzle, R., Fletcher, M., O'Clerigh, J. P. L., et al. (2005). Dispositional optimism and the mechanisms by which it predicts slower disease progression in HIV: Proactive behavior, avoidant coping, and depression. *International Journal of Behavioral Medicine, 12*(2), 86–97; Moskowitz, J. T. (2003). Positive affect predicts lower risk of AIDS mortality. *Psychosomatic Medicine, 65,* 620–626; Segerstrom, S. C., Taylor, S. E., Kemeny, M. E., & Fahey, J. L. (1998). Optimism is associated with mood, coping, and immune change in response to stress. *Journal of Personality and Social Psychology, 74*(5), 1646–1655.

34. Anda, R., Williamson, D. Jones, D., Macera, C., Eaker, E., Glassman, A., & Marks, James. (1993). Depressed affect, hopelessness, and the risk of ischemic heart disease in a cohort of U.S. adults. *Epidemiology, 4*(4), 285–294; Everson, S. A., Goldberg, D. E., Kaplan, G. A., Cohen, R. D., Pukkala, E., Tuomilehto, J., et al. (1996). Hopelessness and risk of mortality and incidence of myocardial infarction and cancer. *Psychosomatic Medicine, 58,* 113–121; Todaro, J. F., Shen, B., Niaura, R., Spiro III, A., & Ward, K. D. (2003). Effect of negative emotions on the frequency of coronary heart disease. *The American Journal of Cardiology, 92,* 901–906.

35. Everson, S. A., Goldberg, D. E., Kaplan, G. A., Cohen, R. D., Pukkala, E., Tuomilehto, J., et al. (1996). Hopelessness and risk of mortality and incidence of myocardial infarction and cancer. *Psychosomatic Medicine, 58*, 113–121; Giltay, E. J., Geleijnse, J. M., Zitman, F. G., Hoestra, T., Schouten, E. G. (2004). Dispositional optimism and all-cause and cardiovascular mortality in a prospective cohort of elderly Dutch men and women. *Archives of General Psychiatry, 61*, 1126–1135; Kubzansky, L. D., Sparrow, D., Vokonas, P., & Kawachi, I. (2001). Is the glass half empty or half full? A prospective study of optimism and coronary heart disease in the normative aging study. *Psychosomatic Medicine, 63*, 910–6; Stern, S. S., Dhanda, R., & Hazuda, H. P. (2001). Hopelessness predicts mortality in older Mexican and European Americans. *Psychosomatic Medicine, 63*, 344–35; Taylor, S. E., Kemeny, M. E., Reed, G. M., Bower, J. E., & Gruenewald, T. L. (2000). Psychological resources, positive illusions, and health. *American Psychologist, 55*(1), 99–109.

36. Brummett, B. H., Helms, M. J., Dahlstrom, G., & Siegler, I. C. (2006). Prediction of all-cause mortality by the Minnesota Multiphasic Personality Inventory Optimism-Pessimism scale scores: Study of a college sample during a 40-year follow-up period. *Mayo Clinic Proceedings, 81*(12), 1541–1544; Maruta, T., Colligan, R. C., Malinchoc, M. & Offord, K. P. (2000). Optimists vs. pessimists: Survival rate among medical patients over a 30-year period. *Mayo Clinic Proceedings, 75*, 140–143.

37. Dello Buono, M., Urciruoli, O., DeLeo, D. (1998). Quality of life and longevity: A study of centenarians. *Age and Aging, 27*, 207–216.

38. Pitkala, K. H., Laakkhonen, M. L., Strandberg, T. A., & Tilvis, R. S. (2004). Positive life orientation as a predictor of 10-year outcome in an aged population. *Journal of Clinical Epidemiology, 57*, 409–414.

39. Seligman, M. (2000). Optimism, pessimism, and mortality. *Mayo Clinic Proceedings, 75*(2), 133–134.

40. Ganguli, M., Dodge, H. H., & Mulsant, B. H. (2002). Rates and predictors of mortality in an aging, rural, community-based cohort. *Archives of General Psychiatry, 59*, 1046–1052; Giltay, E. J., Kamphuis, M. H., Kalmijn, S., Zitman, F. G., & Kromhout, D. (2006). Dispositional optimism and the risk of cardiovascular death. *Archives of General Psychiatry, 166*, 431–436; Penninx, B. W. J. H., Beekman, A. T. F., Honig, A., Deeg, D. J. H., Schoevers, R. A., van Eijk, J. T. M., & van Tilberg, W. (2001). Depression and cardiac mortality. *Archives of General Psychiatry, 58*, 221–227; Penninx, B. W. J. H., Geerlings, S. W., Deeg, D. J. H., van Eijk, J. T. M., van Tilberg, W., & Beekman, A. T. F. (1999). Minor and

major depression and the risk of death in older persons. *Archives of General Psychiatry, 56,* 889–895; Saz, P. & Dewey, M. E. (2001). Depression, depressive symptoms and mortality in persons aged 65 years and over living in the community: A systematic review of the literature. *International Journal of Geriatric Psychiatry, 16,* 622–630.

41. Schulz, R., Beach, S. R., Ives, D. G., Martire, L. M., Ariyo, A. A., & Kop, W. J. (2000). Association between depression and mortality in older adults. *Archives of Internal Medicine, 160,* 1761–1768; Whooley, M. A. & Browner, W. S. (1998). Association between depressive symptoms and mortality in older women. *Archives of Internal Medicine, 158,* 2129–2135.

42. Aspinwall, L. G. & Brunhart, S. M. (1996). Distinguishing optimism from denial: Optimistic beliefs predict attention to health threats. *Personality and Social Psychology Bulletin, 22*(10), 993–1003; Nes, L. S. & Segerstrom, S. C. (2006). Dispositional optimism and coping: A meta-analytic review. *Personality and Social Psychology Review, 10*(3), 235–251.

43. Taylor, S. E., Kemeny, M. E., Reed, G. M., Bower, J. E., & Gruenewald, T. L. (2000). Psychological resources, positive illusions, and health. *American Psychologist, 55*(1), 99–109.

CHAPTER 9

1. Baltes, P. B., Staudinger, U. M., Maercker, A., & Smith, J. (1995). People nominated as wise: A comparative study of wisdom-related knowledge. *Psychology and Aging, 10,* 155–166.

2. Cozolino, L. J. (2017). *The neuroscience of psychotherapy: Building and rebuilding the human brain* (3rd ed). New York: Norton; Ruisel, I. (2005). Wisdom's role in interactions of affects and cognition. *Studia Psychologica, 47,* 277–289; Yang, S.-Y. (2001). Conceptions of wisdom among Taiwanese Chinese. *Journal of Cross-Cultural Psychology, 32,* 662–680.

3. Ochsner, K. N., Beer, J. S., Robertson, E. R., Cooper, J. C., Gabrieli, J. D. E., Kihlstrom, J. F., et al. (2005). The neural correlates of direct and reflected self-knowledge. *NeuroImage, 28,* 797–814.

4. Happé, F. G. E., Winner, E., & Brownell, H. (1998). The getting of wisdom: Theory of mind in old age. *Developmental Psychology, 34,* 358–362.

5. Hashtroudi, S., Johnson, M. K, & Chrosniak, L. D. (1990). Aging and qualitative characteristics of memories for perceived and imagined complex events. *Psychology and Aging, 5,* 119–126.

6. Tentori, K., Osherson, D., Hasher, L., & May, C. (2001). Wisdom and aging: Irrational preferences in college students but not older adults. *Cognition, 81,* B87–B96.

7. Mesulam, M. M. (1987). Involutional and developmental implications of age-related neuronal changes: In search of an engram for wisdom. *Neurobiology of Aging, 8,* 581–583.

8. Knight, R. T., & Grabowecky, M. (1995). Escape from linear time: Prefrontal cortex and conscious experience. In M. S. Gazzaniga (Ed.), *The Cognitive Neurosciences.* Cambridge: MIT Press.

9. Winnicott, D. W. (1958). The capacity to be alone. In D. W. Winnicott (1965), *Maturational processes and the facilitating environment* (pp. 29-36). New York: International Universities Press.

10. Joseph, R. (1996). *Neuropsychiatry, neuropsychology, and clinical neuroscience.* Baltimore: Williams & Wilkins.

11. Dawson, G., Panagiotides, H., Klinger, L. G., & Spieker, S. (1997). Infants of depressed and non-depressed mothers exhibit differences in frontal brain electrical activity during the expressions of negative emotions. *Developmental Psychology, 33,* 650–656.

12. Newberg, A., Alavi, A., Baime, M., Pourdehnad, M., Santanna, J., & Aquili, E. (2001). The measurement of cerebral blood flow during the complex cognitive task of meditation: A preliminary SPECT study. *Psychiatric Research: Neuroimaging Section, 106,* 113–122.

13. Kaasinen, V., Maguire, R. P., Kurki, T., Bruck, A., & Rinne, J. O. (2005). Mapping brain structure and personality in late adulthood. *NeuroImage, 24,* 315–322.

14. Kjaer, T. W., Nowak, M., & Lou, H. C. (2002). Reflective self-awareness and conscious states: PET evidence for a common midline parietofrontal core. *NeuroImage, 17,* 1080–1086; Lou, H. C., Luber, B., Crupain, M., Keenan, J. P., Nowak, M., Kjaer, T. W., et al. (2004). Parietal cortex and representation of the mental self. *Proceedings of the National Academy of Sciences, USA, 101,* 6827–6832.

15. von Bonin, G. (1963). *The evolution of the human brain.* Chicago: University of Chicago Press.

CHAPTER 10

1. Dunbar, R. I. (1996). *Grooming, gossip, and the evolution of language.* Cambridge: Harvard University Press.

2. Arbuckle, T. Y., & Gold, D. P. (1993). Aging, inhibition, and verbosity. *Journal of Gerontology: Psychological Sciences, 48,* P225–P232.

3. Burke, D. M. (1997). Language, aging, and inhibitory deficits: Evaluation of a theory. *Journals of Gerontology, 52B,* 254–264; Hasher, L., Quig, M. B., & May, C. P. (1997). Inhibitory control over no-longer-relevant information: Adult age differences. *Memory and Cognition, 25,* 286–295;

Hashtroudi, S., Johnson, M. K, & Chrosniak, L. D. (1990). Aging and qualitative characteristics of memories for perceived and imagined complex events. *Psychology and Aging, 5,* 119–126.

4. Shewan, C. M., & Henderson, V. L. (1988). Analysis of spontaneous language in the older normal population. *Journal of Communication Disorders, 21,* 139–154.

5. James, L. E., Burke, D. M., Austin, A., & Hulme, E. (1998). Production and perception of "verbosity" in younger and older adults. *Psychology and Aging, 13,* 355–367.

6. Ryan, E. B., See, S. K., Meneer, W. B., & Trovato, D. (1992). Age-based perceptions of language performance among younger and older adults. *Communication Research, 19,* 423–443.

7. Frenkel-Brunswik, E. (1936). Studies in biographical psychology. *Character and Personality, 5,* 1–34.

8. Duvarci, S., & Nader, K. (2004). Characterization of fear memory reconsolidation. *Journal of Neuroscience, 24,* 9269–9275; Nader, K. (2003). Memory traces unbound. *Trends in Neurosciences, 26,* 65–72.

9. Marini, A., Carlomagno, S., Caltagirone, C., & Nocentini, U. (2005). The role played by the right hemisphere in the organization of complex textual structures. *Brain and Language, 93,* 46–54; Shumake, J., Conejo-Jimenez, N., Gonzalez-Pardo, H., & Gonzalez-Lima, F. (2004). Brain differences in newborn rats predisposed to helpless and depressive behavior. *Brain Research, 1030,* 267–276; Tucker, D. M., Luu, P., & Pribram, K. H. (1995). Social and emotional self-regulation. In J. Grafman & K.J. Hoyoak, (Eds.), *Structure and functions of the human prefrontal cortex,* (pp. 213–239). New York: New York Academy of Sciences.

10. Faust, M., & Weisper, S. (2000). Understanding metaphoric sentences in the two cerebral hemispheres. *Brain and Cognition, 43,* 186–191.

11. Bluck, S., & Glück, J. (2004). Making things better and learning a lesson: Experiencing wisdom across the lifespan. *Journal of Personality, 72,* 543–572; McAdams, D. P., Reynolds, J., Lewis, M., Patten, A. H., & Bowman, P. J. (2001). When bad things turn good and good things turn bad: Sequences of redemption and contamination in life narrative and their relation to psychosocial adaptation in midlife adults and in students. *Personality and Social Psychology Bulletin, 27,* 474–485.

12. Beeghly, M., & Cicchetti, D, (1994). Child maltreatment, attachment, and the self-system: Emergence of an internal state lexicon in toddlers at high social risk. *Development and Psychopathology, 6,* 5–30; Fonagy, P., Leigh, T., Steele, M., Steele, H., Kennedy, R., Mattoon, G., et al. (1996). The relation of attachment status, psychiatric classification, and

response to psychotherapy. *Journal of Consulting and Clinical Psychology, 64,* 22–31; Main, M., Kaplan, N., & Cassidy, J. (1985). Security in infancy, childhood, and adulthood: A move to the level of representation. In I. Bretherton & E. Waters (Eds.), *Growing points of attachment theory and research. Monographs of the Society for Research in Child Development, 50,* 66–104.

13. Christensen, A. J., Edwards, D. L., Wiebe, J. S., Benotsch, E. G., McKelvey, L., Andrews, M., et al. (1996). Effect of verbal self-disclosure on natural killer cell activity: Moderating influence of cynical hostility. *Psychosomatic Medicine, 58,* 150–155; Esterling, B. A., Antoni, M. H., Fletcher, M. A., Margulies, S., & Schneiderman, N. (1994). Emotional disclosure through writing or speaking modulates latent Epstein-Barr virus antibody titers. *Journal of Consulting and Clinical Psychology, 62,* 130–140; Pennebaker, J. W., Kiecolt-Glaser, J. K., & Glaser, R. (1988). Disclosure of traumas and immune function: Health implications for psychotherapy. *Journal of Consulting and Clinical Psychology, 56,* 239–245.

14. Fonagy, P., Steele, M., Steele, H., Moran, G. S., & Higgitt, A. C. (1991). The capacity to understand mental states: The reflective self in parent and child and its significance for security of attachment. *Infant Mental Health Journal, 12,* 201–218.

15. Fonagy, P., Leigh, T., Steele, M., Steele, H., Kennedy, R., Mattoon, G., et al. (1996). The relation of attachment status, psychiatric classification, and response to psychotherapy. *Journal of Consulting and Clinical Psychology, 64,* 22–31.

CHAPTER 11

1. Aiello, L. C., & Wells, J. C. K. (2002). Energetics and the evolution of the genus homo. *Annual Review of Anthrolpology, 31,* 323–338; Finch, C. E., & Stanford, C. B. (2004). Meat-adaptive genes and the evolution of slower aging in humans. *Quarterly Review of Biology, 79,* 3–50.

2. Leonard, W. R., Robertson, M. L., Snodgrass, J. J., & Kuzawa, C. W. (2003). Metabolic correlates of hominid brain evolution. *Comparative Biochemistry and Physiology: Part A, 136,* 5–15.

3. Aiello, L. C., & Wheeler, P. (1995). The expensive-tissue hypothesis: The brain and the digestive system in human and primate evolution. *Current Anthropology, 36,* 199–221.

4. Galli, R. L., Shukitt-Hale, B., Youdim, K. A., & Joseph, J. A. (2002). Fruit polyphenolics and brain aging: Nutritional interventions targeting age-related neuronal and behavioral deficits. *Annals of the New York*

Academy of Sciences, 959, 128–132; Lau, F. C., Shukitt-Hale, & Joseph, J. A. (2005). The beneficial effects of fruit polyphenols on brain aging. Neurobiology of Aging 268, S128–S132; Lau, F. C., Bielinski, D. F., & Joseph J. A. (2007). Inhibitory effects of blueberry extract on the production of inflammatory mediators in lipopolysaccharide-activated BV2 microglia. Journal of Neuroscience Research, 85(5), 1010–1017.

5. Duthie, S. J., Whalley, L. J., Collins, A. R., Leaper, S., Berger, K., & Deary, I. J. (2002). Homocysteine, b vitamin status, and cognitive function in the elderly. The American Journal of Clinical Nutrition, 75, 908–913; Kruman, I. I., Kumaravel, T. S., Lohani, A., Pedersen, W. A., Cutler, R. G., Kruman, Y., Haughey, N., Lee, J., Evans, M., & Mattson, M. P. (2002). Folic acid deficiency and homocysteine impair DNA repair in hippocampal neurons and sensitize them to amyloid toxicity in experimental models of alzheimer's disease. Journal of Neuroscience, 22(5), 1752–1762; Mattson, M. P. (2003). Gene-diet interactions in brain aging and neurodegenerative disorders. Annals of Internal Medicine, 139(5), 441–444; Mattson, M. P., Kruman, I. I., &Duan, W. (2002). Folic acid and homocysteine in age-related disease. Ageing Research Reviews, 1, 95–111.

6. Uauy, R. & Dangour, A. D. (2006). Nutrition in brain development and aging: role of essential fatty acids. Nutrition Reviews, 64(5), S24–S33.

7. Franco, O. H., Burger, H., Lebrun, C. E. I., Peeters, P. H. M., Lamberts, S. W. J., Grobbee, D. E., et al. (2005). Higher dietary intake of lignans is associated with better cognitive performance in postmenopausal women. The Journal of Nutrition, 135, 1190–1195; Zhao, L., Chen, Q., Brinton, R. D. (2002). Neuroprotective and neurotrophic efficacy of phytoestrogens in cultured hippocampal neurons. Experimental Biology and Medicine, 22(7), 509–519.

8. Swain, R. A., Harris, A. B., Wiener, E. C., Dutka, M. V., Morris, H. D., Theien, B. E., et al. (2003). Prolonged exercise induces angiogenesis and increases cerebral blood volume in primary motor cortex of the rat. Neuroscience, 117, 1037–1046.

9. Cotman, C. W., & Berchtold, N. C. (2002). Exercise: A behavioral intervention to enhance brain health and plasticity. Trends in Neurosciences, 25, 295–301.

10. Hobson, J. A. (1989). Sleep. New York: Scientific American Library.

11. Cirelli, C. (2005). A molecular window on sleep: Changes in gene expression between sleep and wakefulness. Neuroscientist, 11, 63–74; Ding, J., Gip, P. T., Franken, P., Lomas, L., O'Hara, B. F. (2004). A proteomic analysis in brain following sleep deprivation suggests a gen-

eralized decrease in abundance for many proteins. *Sleep 27S*, A391; Nakanishi, H., Sun, Y., Nakamura, R. K., Mori, K., Ito, M., Suda, S. et al. (1997). Positive Correlations between cerebral protein synthesis rates and deep sleep in macaca mulatta. *European Journal of Neuroscience*, 9(2), 271–279; Ribeiro, S., Goyal, V., Mello, C. V.,& Pavlides, C. (1999). Brain gene expression during REM sleep depends on prior waking experience. *Learning and Memory*, 6, 500 – 508; Taishi, P., Sanchez, C., Wang, Y., Fang, J., Harding, J. W., Krueger, J. M. (2001). Conditions that affect sleep alter the expression of molecules associated with synaptic plasticity. *American Journal of Physiology. Regulatory, Integrative and Comparative Physiology*, 281(3), R839–R845.

12. Buzsaki, G. (1998). Memory consolidation during sleep: a neurophysiological perspective. *Journal of Sleep Research, 7, Suppl. 1*, 17 – 23; Frank, M. G., Issa, N. P., Stryker, M. P. (2001). Sleep enhances plasticity in the developing visual cortex. *Neuron, 30*, 275–287; Macquet, P. (2001). The role of sleep in learning and memory. *Science*, 294(5544), 1048 – 1052; Walker, M. P., & Stickgold, R.(2004). Sleep-dependent learning and memory consolidation. *Neuron, 44*, 121–133; Walker, M. P.,& Stickgold, R. (2006). Sleep, memory, and plasticity. *Annual Review of Psychology, 57*, 139–166.

13. Gais, S., Plihal, W., Wagner, U., Born, J. (2000). Early sleep triggers memory for early visual discrimination skills. *Nature Neuroscience, 3(12)*, 1335 – 1339; Karni, A., Tanne, D., Rubenstein, B. S., Askenasy, J. J. M., & Sagi, D. (1994). Dependence on REM sleep of overnight improvement of a perceptual skill. *Science, 265*, 679–682; Mednick, S. C., Nakayama, K., Cantero, J. L., Atienza, M., Levin, A. A., Pathak, N., Stickgold, R. (2002). The restorative effect of naps on perceptual deterioration *Nature Neuroscience, 5(7)*, 677–681; Smith, C. (1995). Sleep states and memory processes. *69*, 137–145; Stickgold, R., James, L., Hobson, J. A. (2000). Visual discrimination learning requires sleep after training. *Nature Neuroscience, 3(12)*, 1237–1238; Walker, M. P., Stickgold, R., Alsop, D., Gaab, N., Schlaug, G. (2005). Sleep-dependent motor memory plasticity in the human brain. *Neuroscience, 133*, 911–917.

14. Gais, S., Lucas, B., Born, J. (2006). Sleep after learning aids memory recall. *Learning and Memory, 13*, 259 – 262; Wagner, U., Gais, S., Born, J. (2001). Emotional memory formation is enhanced across sleep intervals with high amounts of rapid eye movement sleep. *Learning and Memory, 8*, 112–119.

15. Mazzarello, P. (2000). What dreams may come? The scientific benefits of eating cheese before bedtime. *Nature, 408*, 523.

16. Wagner, U., Gais, S., Haider, H., Verleger, R., & Born, J. (2004). Sleep inspires insight. *Nature, 427,* 352–355.
17. Ancoli-Israel, S. & Cooke, J. R. (2005). Prevalence and comorbidity of insomnia and effect on functioning in elderly populations. *Journal of American Geriatrics Society, 53,* S264 – S271; Ancoli-Israel, S., Poceta, J. S., Stepnowsky, C., Martin, J., & Gehrman, P. (1997). Identification and treatment of sleep problems in the elderly. *Sleep Medicine Reviews,* 1(1), 3 – 17. Brabbins, C. J., Dewey, M. E., Copeland, J. R. M., Davidson, I. A., McWIlliam, C., Saunders, P. et al. (1993). Insomnia in the elderly: prevalence, gender differences and relationships with morbidity and mortality. *International Journal of Geriatric psychiatry, 8,* 473–480; Floyd, J., Medler, S. M., Ager, J. W., & Janisse, J. J. (2000). Age-related changes in initiation and maintenance of sleep: a meta-analysis. *Research in Nursing & Health, 23,* 106–117; Neubauer, D. N. (1999). Sleep problems in the elderly. *American Family Physician, 59*(9), 2551; Wolkove, N., Elkholy, O., Baltzan, M., & Palayew, M. (2007). Sleep and aging: 1. Sleep disorders commonly found in older people. *Canadian Medical Association Journal, 176*(9), 1299–1304.
18. Durmer, J. S., & Dinges, D. F. (2005). Neurocognitive consequences of sleep deprivation. *Seminars in Neurology, 25,* 117–129.
19. Brabbins, C. J., Dewey, M. E., Copeland, J. R. M., Davidson, I. A., McWIlliam, C., Saunders, P. et al. (1993). Insomnia in the elderly: prevalence, gender differences and relationships with morbidity and mortality. *International Journal of Geriatric psychiatry, 8,* 473–480; Foley, D. J., Monjan, A. A., Brown, S. L., Simonsick, E. M., Wallace, R. B., & Blazer, D. G. (1995). Sleep complaints among elderly persons: an epidemiologic study of three communities. *Sleep, 18,* 425–432; Giron, M. S. T., Forsell, V., Bernsten, C., Thorslund, M., Winblad, B., & Fastbom, J. (2002). Sleep problems in a very old population: drug use and clinical correlates. *The Journals of Gerontology, 57A*(4), M236 – M240; Monane, M. (1992). Insomnia in the elderly. *Journal of Clinical Psychiatry, 53*(Supp.), 23–28.
20. Ancoli-Israel, S. & Cooke, J. R. (2005). Prevalence and comorbidity of insomnia and effect on functioning in elderly populations. *Journal of American Geriatrics Society, 53,* S264 – S271.
21. Wolkove, N., Elkholy, O., Baltzan, M., & Palayew, M. (2007). Sleep and aging: 1. Sleep disorders commonly found in older people. *Canadian Medical Association Journal, 176*(9), 1299–1304.
22. Ancoli-Israel, S. & Cooke, J. R. (2005). Prevalence and comorbidity of insomnia and effect on functioning in elderly populations. *Journal of*

American Geriatrics Society, 53, S264 – S271; Ancoli-Israel, S., Poceta, J. S., Stepnowsky, C., Martin, J., & Gehrman, P. (1997). Identification and treatment of sleep problems in the elderly. *Sleep Medicine Reviews, 1*(1), 3 – 17; Van Someren, E. J. W. (2000). Circadian and sleep disturbances in the elderly. *Experimental Gerontology, 35*, 1229–1237.

23. van Coevorden, A., Mockel, J., Laurent, E., Kerkhofs, M., L'Hermite-Balériaux, M., Decoster, C., et al. (1991). Neuroendocrine rhythms and sleep in aging men. *American Journal of Physiology, 260*, E651–E661; Van Someren, E. J. W. (2000). Circadian and sleep disturbances in the elderly. *Experimental Gerontology, 35*, 1229–1237.

24. Fetveit, A., Skjerve, A., & Bjorvatn, B. (2003). Bright light treatment improves sleep in institutionalized elderly – an open trial. *International Journal of Geriatric Psychiatry, 18*, 520–526; Martin, J., Shochat, T., & Ancoli-Israel, S. (2000). Assessment and treatment of sleep disturbances in older adults. *Clinical Psychology Review, 20*(6), 783–805; Morin, C. M., Mimeault, V., & Gagne, A. (1999). Nonpharmacological treatment of late-life insomnia. *Journal of Psychosomatic Research, 46*(2), 103–116.

25. Ancoli-Israel, S., Poceta, J. S., Stepnowsky, C., Martin, J., & Gehrman, P. (1997). Identification and treatment of sleep problems in the elderly. *Sleep Medicine Reviews, 1*(1), 3 – 17; Morin, C. M., Kowatch, R. A., Barry, T., & Walton, E. (1993). Cognitive-behavior therapy for late-life insomnia. *Journal of Consulting and Clinical Psychology, 61*, 137–146; Morin, C. M., Colecchi, C., Stone, J., Sood, R., & Brink, D. (1999). Behavioral and pharmacological treatments for late-life insomnia: A randomized controlled trial. *Journal of the American Medical Association, 281*, 991–999; Shochat, T., Loredo, J., & Ancoli-Israel, S. (2007). Sleep disorders in the elderly. *Current Treatment Options in Neurology, 3*, 19–36; Wolkove, N., Elkholy, O., Baltzan, M., & Palayew, M. (2007b). Sleep and aging: 2. Management of sleep disorders in older people. *Canadian Medical Association Journal, 176*(10), 1449–1454.

26. United Nations Department of Economic and Social Affairs Population Division. (1998). *World Population Prospects* (1998 Revision). New York, NY: Author.

27. Bernstein, A. M., Willcox, B. J., Tamaki, H., Kunishima, N., Suzuki, M., Willcox, D. C. & et al. (2004). First autopsy study of an Okinawan centenarian: Absence of many age-related diseases. *Journal of Gerontology: MEDICAL SCIENCES, 59A*(11), 1195–1199; Franceschi, C., & Bonafè, M. (2003). Centenarians as a model for healthy aging. *Biochemical Society Transactions, 31*, 457–461; Koenig, R. (2001). Sardinia's mys-

terious male methuselahs. *Science, 291*, 2074–2076; Perls, T. T., Kunke, L. M., Puca, A. A. (2002). The genetics of exceptional human longevity. *Journal of Molecular Neuroscience, 19*, 233–238.

28. Rowe, J. W., & Kahn, R. L. (1997). Successful aging. *The Gerontologist, 37*(4), 433–440.

29. Andersen-Ranberg, K., Schroll, M., & Jeune, B. (2001). Healthy centenarians do not exist, but autonomous centenarians do: A population based study of morbidity among Danish centenarians. *Journal of the American Geriatric Society, 49*, 900–908; Gondo, Y., Hirose, N., & Arai, Y. (2006). Functional status of centenarians in Tokyo: Developing better phenotypes of exceptional longevity. *Journals of Gerontology: Medical Sciences, 61A*(3), 305–310; Martin, P., Rott, C., Hagberg, B., & Morgan, K. (2000). Centenarians: Autonomy versus dependence in the oldest old. Springer, New York Berlin Heidelberg; Motta, M., Bennati, E., Ferlito, L., Malguarnera, M., & Motta, L. (2005). Successful aging in centenarians: Myths and reality. *Archives of Gerontology and Geriatrics, 40*, 241–251.

30. Fries, J. F., Koop, C. E., Sokolov, J., Beadle, C. E., & Wright, D. (1998). Beyond health promotion: reducing need and demand for medical care. *Health Affairs, 17*(2), 70–84; Hitt, R., Young-Xu, Y., Silver, M. & Perls, T. (1999). Centenarians: The older you get, the healthier you have been. *The Lancet, 354*, 652; Willcox, D. C., Willcox, B. J., Shimajir, S., Kurechi, S., & Suzuki, M. (2007). Aging gracefully: A retrospective analysis of functional status in Okinawan centenarians. *American Journal of Geriatric Psychiatry, 15*(3), 252–256.

31. Poon, L. W., Clayton, G. M., Martin, P., Johnson, M. A., Courtenay, B. C., Sweaney, A. L., et al. (1992). The Georgia Centenarian Study. *International Journal of Aging & Human Development, 34*, 1–7.

32. Adkins, F., Martin, P., & Poon, L. W. (1996). Personality traits and states as predictors of subjective well-being in centenarians, octogenarians, and sexagenarians. *Psychology and Aging, 11*(3), 408–416; Martin, P., DaRosa, F., Siegler, I. C., Davey, A., MacDonald, M., & Poon, L. W. (2006). Personality and longevity: Findings from the Georgia Centenarian Study. *Age, 28*, 343–352; Masui, Y., Gondo, Y., Inagaki, H., & Hirose, N. (2006). Do personality characteristics predict longevity? Findings from the Tokyo Centenarian Study. *Age, 28*, 353–361; Mroczek, D. K., Spiro, A., III, & Griffin P.W. (2006). Personality and aging. In J. E. Birren & K. W. Schaie (Eds.), *Handbook of the psychology of aging* (6th ed.) (pp. 363–377). Amsterdam: Elsevier; Samuelsson, S. M., Alfredson, B. B., Hagberg, B., Sammuelsson, G., Nordbeck, B., Brun,

A., et al. (1997). The Swedish Centenarian Study: A multidisciplinary study of five consecutive cohorts at the age of 100. *International Journal of Aging and Human Development, 45,* 223–253; Shimonaka, Y., Nakazato, K., & Homma, K. (1996). Personality, longevity, and successful aging among Tokyo Metropolitan centenarians. *International Journal of Aging and Human Development, 42,* 173–187.

33. Adkins, F., Martin, P., & Poon, L. W. (1996). Personality traits and states as predictors of subjective well-being in centenarians, octogenarians, and sexagenarians. *Psychology and Aging, 11*(3), 408–416; Martin, P., DaRosa, F., Siegler, I. C., Davey, A., MacDonald, M., & Poon, L. W. (2006). Personality and longevity: Findings from the Georgia Centenarian Study. *Age, 28,* 343–352; Masui, Y., Gondo, Y., Inagaki, H., & Hirose, N. (2006). Do personality characteristics predict longevity? Findings from the Tokyo Centenarian Study. *Age, 28,* 353–361.

34. Dello Buono, M., Urciruoli, O., DeLeo, D. (1998). Quality of life and longevity: A study of centenarians. *Age and Aging, 27,* 207–216.

CHAPTER 12

1. Baltes, P. B., & Lindenberger, U. (1997). Emergence of a powerful connection between sensory and cognitive functions across the adult life span: A new window to the study of cognitive aging? *Psychology and Aging, 12,* 12–21; Lindenberger, U., & Baltes, P. B. (1997). Intellectual functioning in old and very old age: Cross-sectional results from the Berlin aging study. *Psychology and Aging, 12,* 410–432; Tabbarah, M., Crimmins, E. M., & Seeman, T. E. (2002). The relationship between cognitive and physical performance: MacArthur studies of successful aging. *Journal of Gerontology: Medical Sciences, 57A,* M228–M235.

2. Schaie, K. W. (1989). Perceptual speed in adulthood: Cross-sectional and longitudinal studies. *Psychology and Aging, 4,* 443–453.

3. Laurienti, P. J., Burdette, J. H., Maldjian, J. A., Wallace, M. T. (2005). Enhanced multisensory integration in older adults. *Neurobiology of Aging* (In Press); Skipper, J. I., Nusbaum, H. C., & Small, S. L. (2005). Listening to talking faces: Motor cortical activation during speech perception. *NeuroImage, 25,* 76–89.

4. Nusbaum, N. J. (1999). Aging and sensory senescence. *Southern Medical Journal, 92,* 267–275.

5. de Rekeneire, N., Visser, M., Peila, R., Nevitt, M. C., Cauley, J. A., Tylavsky, F. A., et al. (2003). Is a fall just a fall: Correlates of falling in healthy older persons. The health, aging and body composition study. *Journal of the American Geriatrics Society, 51,* 841–846.

6. Francis, D. D., Champagne, F. A., Liu, D. & Meaney, M. J. (1999). Maternal care, gene expression, and the development of individual differences in stress reactivity. *Annals of New York Academy of Sciences, 896*, 66–84; Olausson, H., Lamarre, Y., Backlund, H., Morin, C., Wallin, B. G., Starck, G., et al. (2002). Unmyelinated tactile afferents signal touch and project to insular cortex. *Nature Neuroscience, 5*, 900–904; Rolls, E. T., O'Doherty, J., Kringelbach, M.L., Francis, S., Bowtell, R., & McGlone, F. (2003). Representations of pleasant and painful touch in the human orbitofrontal and cingulate cortices. *Cerebral Cortex, 13*, 308–317.

7. Berns, G. S., McClure, S. M., Pagnoni, G., & Montague, P.R. (2001). Predictability modulates human brain response to reward. *Journal of Neuroscience, 21*, 2793–2798; Fiorillo, C. D., Tobler, P. N., & Schultz, W. (2003). Discrete coding of reward probability and uncertainty by dopamine neurons. *Science, 299*, 1898–1902; Mirenowicz, J., & Schultz, W. (1994). Importance of unpredictability for reward responses in primate dopamine neurons. *Journal of Neurophysiology, 72*, 1024–1027.

8. Knox, S. S., & Uvnäs-Moberg, K. (1998). Social isolation and cardiovascular disease: An atherosclerotic pathway? *Psychoneuroendocrinology, 23*, 877–890; Weller, A., & Feldman, R. (2003). Emotion regulation and touch in infants: The role of cholecystokinin and opioids. *Peptides, 24*, 779–788.

9. Anderson, G. C. (1991). Current knowledge about skin-to-skin (kangaroo) care for preterm infants. *Journal of Perinatology, 11*, 216–226; Bergman, N. J., Linley, L. L., & Fawcus, S. R. (2004). Randomized controlled trial of skin-to-skin contact from birth versus conventional incubator for physiological stabilization in 1200- to 2199- gram newborns. *Acta Paediatrica, 93*, 779–785; Field, T. M., Gizzle, N., Scafidi, F., Abrams, S., Richardson, S., Kuhn, C., et al. (1996). Massage therapy for infants of depressed mothers. *Infant Behavior and Development, 19*, 107–112; Ottenbacher, K. J., Muller, L., Brandt, D., Heintzelman, A., Hojem, P., & Sharpe, P. (1987). The effectiveness of tactile stimulation as a form of early intervention: A quantitative evaluation. *The Journal of Developmental and Behavioral Pediatrics, 8*, 68–76.

10. Anisfeld, E., Casper, V., Nozyce, M., & Cunningham, N. (1990). Does infant carrying promote attachment? An experimental study of the effects of increased physical contact on the development of attachment. *Child Development, 61*(5), 1617–1627; Fleming, A. S., Kraemer, G. W., Gonzalez, A., Lovic, V., Rees, S., & Melo, A. (2002). Mothering begets mothering: the transmission of behavior and its neurobiology across generations. *Pharmacology, Biochemistry and Behavior, 73*, 61–75; Levine,

S., Haltmeyer, G. C., Karas, G. G., & Denenberg, V. H. (1967). Physiological and behavioral effects of infantile stimulation. *Physiology and Behavior, 2*, 55–59; Meaney, M. J., Aitken, D. H., Viau, V., Sharma, S., & Sarrieau, A. (1989). Neonatal handling alters adrenocortical negative feedback sensitivity and hippocampal type II glucocorticoid receptor binding in the rat. *Neuroendocrinology, 50*, 597–604.

11. Liu, D., Diorio, J., Tannenbaum, B., Caldji, C., Francis, D., Freedman, A., et al. (1997). Maternal care, hippocampal glucocorticoid receptors, and hypothalamic-pituitary-adrenal responses to stress. *Science, 277*, 1659–1662; Meaney, M. J., Diorio, J., Francis, D., Weaver, S., Yau, J., Chapman, K., & Seckl, J. R. (2000). Postnatal handling increases the expression of CAMP-inducible transcription factors in the rat hippocampus: The effects of thyroid hormones and serotonin. *Journal of Neuroscience, 20*, 3926–3935; Sapolsky, R. M. (1990). Stress in the wild. *Scientific American, 262*(1), 116–123; Smythe, J. W., Rowe, W. B., & Meaney, M. J. (1994). Neonatal handling alters serotonin (5-HT) turnover and 5-HT2 receptor binding in selected brain regions: Relationship to the handling effect on glucocorticoid receptor expression. *Developmental Brain Research, 80*, 183–189.

12. Goodfellow, L. M. (2003). The effects of therapeutic back massage on psychophysiologic variables and immune function in spouses of patients with cancer. *Nursing Research, 52*, 318–328; Hernandez-Reif, M., Ironson, G., Field, T., Hurley, J., Katz, G., Diego, M., et al. (2004). Breast cancer patients have improved immune and neuroendocrine functions following massage therapy. *Journal of Psychosomatic Research, 57*, 45–52; Lund, I., Long-Chuan, Y., Uvnäs-Moberg, K., Wang, J., Yu, C., Kurosawa, M., et al (2002). Repeated massage-like stimulation induces long-term effects on nociception: Contribution on oxytocinergic mechanisms. *European Journal of Neuroscience, 16*, 330–338.

13. Diego, M. A., Field, T., Hernandez-Reif, M., Shaw, K., Friedman, L., & Ironson, G. (2001). HIV adolescents show improved immune function following massage therapy. *International Journal of Neuroscience, 106*, 35–45; Diego, M. A., Field, T., Hernandez-Reif, M., Shaw, J. A., Rothe, E. M., Castellanos, D., et al. (2002). Aggressive adolescents benefit from massage therapy. *Adolescence, 37*, 597–607; Field, T. (2002). Violence and touch deprivation in adolescents. *Adolescence, 37*, 735–749; Jones, N. A., & Field, T. (1999). Massage and music therapies attenuate frontal EEG asymmetry in depressed adolescents. *Adolescence, 34*, 529–534; Remington, R. (2002). Calming music and hand massage with agitated elderly. *Nursing Research, 51*, 317–323.

14. Bush, E. (2001). The use of human touch to improve the well-being of older adults. *Journal of Holistic Nursing*, 19, 256–270.
15. Field, T. M. (1997). The treatment of depressed mothers and their infants. In L. Murry & P. J. Cooper (Eds.), *Postpartum depression and child development*. New York: The Guilford Press; Field, T. (2000). Infant massage therapy. In C. H. Zeanah, Jr. (Ed.), *Handbook of infant mental health* (2nd ed., pp. 494–500). New York: Guilford Press.
16. Field, T. M., Gizzle, N., Scafidi, F., Abrams, S., Richardson, S., Kuhn, C., et al. (1996). Massage therapy for infants of depressed mothers. *Infant Behavior and Development*, 19, 107–112.
17. Onozawa, K., Glover, V., Adams, D., Modi, N., & Kumar, R. C. (2001). Infant massage improves mother-infant interactions for mothers with postnatal depression. *Journal of Affective Disorders*, 63, 201–207.
18. Allman, J., & Brothers, L. (1994). Faces, fear, and the amygdala. *Nature*, 372, 613–614; Machne, X., & Segundo, J. P. (1956). Unitary responses to afferent volleys in amygdaloid complex. *Journal of Neurophysiology*, 19, 232–240.
19. Allen, K. M., Blascovich, J., Tomaka, J., & Kelsey, R. M. (1991). Presence of human friends and pet dogs as moderators of autonomic responses to stress in women. *Journal of Personality and Social Psychology*, 61(4), 582–589; Irani, S., Mahler, C., Goetzmann, L., Russi, E. W., & Boehler, A. (2006). Lung transplant recipients holding companion animals: Impact on physical health and quality of life. *American Journal of Transplantation*, 6, 404–411; McNicholas, J., Gilbey, A., Rennie, A., Ahmedzai, S., Dono, J.-A., & Ormerod, E. (2005). Pet ownership and human health: A brief review of evidence and issues. *BMJ*, 331(7527), 1252–1254.
20. Dembicki, D., & Anderson, J. (1996). Pet ownership may be a factor in improved health of the elderly. *Journal of Nutrition for the Elderly*, 15(3), 15–31; Friedmann, E., Katcher, A. H., Lynch, J. J., & Thomas, S. A. (1980). Animal companions and one-year survival of patients after discharge from a coronary care unit. *Public Health Reports*, 95(4), 307–312; Garrity, T. F., Stallones, L., Marx, M. B., & Johnson, T. P. (1989). Pet ownership and attachment as supportive factors in the health of the elderly. *Anthrozoos*, 3(1), 35-44.
21. Pearce, J. M. S. (2004). Some neurological aspects of laughter. *European Neurology*, 52, 169–171.
22. Bennett, M. P. & Lengacher, C. A. (2006). Humor and laughter may influence health. I. History and background. *Evidence-based Complementary and Alternative Medicine*, 3(1), 61–63; Bennett, M. P. & Lengacher, C. A.

(2006). Humor and laughter may influence health. II. Complementary therapies and humor in a clinical populations. *Evidence-based Complementary and Alternative Medicine, 3*(2), 187–190; Berk, R. A. (2001). The active ingredients in humor: Psychophysiological benefits and risks for older adults. *Educational Gerontology, 27*, 323–9; Takahashi, K., Iwase, M., Yamashita, K., Tatsumoto, Y., Ue, H., Kuratsune, H. et al. (2001). The elevation of natural killer cell activity induced by laughter in a crossover designed study. *International Journal of Molecular Medicine, 8*, 645–650; Ziegler, J. (1995). Immune system may benefit from ability to laugh. *Journal of the National Cancer Institute, 87*(5), 342–343.

23. Hayashi, T., Urayama, O., Kawai, K., Hayashi, K., Iwanaga, S. Ohta, M., Saito, T. et al. (2006). Laughter regulates gene expression in patients with Type 2 diabetes. *Psychotherapy and Psychosomatics, 75*, 62–65.

24. Berk, L. S., Felten, D. L., Tan, S. A., Bittman, B. B., & Westengard, J. (2001). Modulation of neuroimmune parameters during the eustress of humor-associated mirthful laughter. *Alternative Therapies, 7*(2), 62–76; Mobbs, D., Greicius, M. D., Abdel-Azim, E., Menon, V., & Reiss, A. L. (2003). Humor modulates the mesolimbic reward centers. *Neuron, 40*, 1041–1048.

25. Freud, S. (1960). *Jokes and their relation to the unconscious.* New York: Norton

26. Christie, W. & Moore, C. (2004). The impact of humor on patients with cancer. *Clinical Journal of Oncology Nursing, 9*(2), 211–9.

27. Solomon, J. C. (1996). Humor and aging well: A laughing matter or a matter of laughing? *American Behavioral Scientist, 39*(3), 249–271; Westburg, N. G. (2003). Hope, laughter, and humor in residents and staff at an assisted living facility. *Journal of Mental Health Counseling, 25*(1), 16–32.

28. Adamle, K. N. & Ludwick, R. (2005). Humor in hospice care: Who, where, and how much? *American Journal of Hospice & Palliative Medicine, 22*(4), 287–290.

29. Yoder, M. A. & Haude, R. H. (1995). Sense of humor and longevity: Older adults' self-ratings compared with ratings for deceased siblings. *Psychological Reports, 76*, 945–946.

30. Baumeister, R. F., & Leary, M. R. (1995). The need to belong: desire for interpersonal attachments as a fundamental human motivation. *Psychological Bulletin, 117*, 497–529.

31. Bradshaw, G. A., Schore, A. N., Brown, J. L., Poole, J. H., & Moss, C. J. (2005). Elephant breakdown. *Nature, 433*, 807.

32. Baumeister, R. F., & Leary, M. R. (1995). The need to belong: desire for

interpersonal attachments as a fundamental human motivation. *Psychological Bulletin, 117,* 497–529.

33. Kiecolt-Glaser, J. K., McGuire, L., Robles, T. F., & Glaser, R. (2002). Psychoneuroimmunology and psychosomatic medicine: Back to the future. *Psychosomatic Medicine, 64,* 15–28.

34. Cohen, S., & Wills, T. A. (1985). Stress, social support, and the buffering hypothesis. *Psychological Bulletin, 98,* 310–357.

35. Lepore, S. J., Allen, K. A. M., & Evans, G. W. (1993). Social support lowers cardiovascular reactivity to an acute stressor. *Psychosomatic Medicine, 55,* 518–524; Sachser, N., Dürschlag, M., & Hirzel, D. (1998). Social relationships and the management of stress. *Psychoneuroendocrinology, 23,* 891–904.

36. Edens, J. L., Larkin, K. T., & Abel, J. L. (1992). The effect of social support and physical touch on cardiovascular reactions to mental stress. *Journal of Psychosomatic Research, 36,* 371–381; Gerin, W., Pieper, C., Levy, R., & Pickering, T. G. (1992). Social support in social interaction: A moderator of cardiovascular reactivity. *Psychosomatic Medicine, 54,* 324–336; Kamarck, T. W., Manuck, S. B., & Jennings, J. R. (1990). Social support reduces cardiovascular reactivity to psychological challenge: A laboratory model. *Psychosomatic Medicine, 52,* 42–58; Spitzer, S. B., Llabre, M. M., Ironson, G. H., Gellman, M. D., & Schneiderman, N. (1992). The influence of social situations on ambulatory blood pressure. *Psychosomatic Medicine, 54,* 79–86.

37. Berkman, L. F. (1995). The role of social relations in health promotion. *Psychosomatic Medicine, 57,* 245–254.

38. Cobb, S. (1976). Social support as a moderator of life stress. *Psychosomatic Medicine, 38,* 300–314; Levenson, R. W., Carstensen, L. L., & Gottman, J. M. (1994). The influence of age and gender on affect, physiology, and their interrelations: A study of long-term marriages. *Journal of Personality and Social Psychology, 67,* 56–68.

39. Cohen, S. (2004). Social relationships and health. *American Psychologist,* 59676–684; Rowe, J. W., & Kahn, R. L. (1998). *Successful aging.* New York: Dell Publishing.

40. Cacioppo, J. T., & Berntson, G. G. (2002). Social neuroscience. In J. T. Cacioppo, G. G. Berntson, R. Adolphs, C. S. Carter, R. J. Davidson, M. McClintock, et al. (Eds.) *Foundations in social neuroscience* (pp.3–10). Cambridge, MA: MIT Press; House, J. S., Landis, K. R., & Umberson, D. (1988). Social relationships and health. *Science, 241*(4865), 540–545; Thomas, P. D., Goodwin, J. M., & Goodwin, J. S. (1985). Effect of social support on stress-related changes in cholesterol level, uric

Notes

acid level, and immune function in an elderly sample. *American Journal of Psychiatry, 142,* 735–737; Uchino, B. N., Cacioppo, J. T., & Kiecolt-Glaser, J. K. (1996). The relationship between social support and physiological processes: A review with emphasis on underlying mechanisms and implications for health. *Psychological Bulletin, 119*(3), 488–531.

41. Berkman, L. F., & Syme, S. L. (1979). Social networks, host resistance, and mortality: A nine-year follow-up study of Alameda County residents. *American Journal of Epidemiology, 109,* 186–204.

42. Ahituv, A., & Lerman, R. I. (2005, July). *How do marital status, wage rates, and work commitment interact?* (IZA DP No. 1688). Bonn, Germany: Institute for the Study of Labor; Antonovics, K., & Town, R. (2003). *Are all the good men married? Uncovering the sources of the marital wage premium* (Paper 2003'15). San Diego, CA: University of California San Diego, Department of Economics; Bardasi, E., & Taylor, M. (2005, February). Marriage and wages. *Working Papers of the Institute for Social and Economic Research,* paper 20055-1. Colchester: University of Essex.

43. Nock, S. L. (2005). Marriage as a public issue. *The Future of Children, 15(2),* 13–32.

44. Bonn, Germany: Institute for the Study of Labor; Light, A. (2004). Gender differences in the marriage and cohabitation income premium. *Demography, 41*(2), 263–284. Ginther, D. K., & Zovodny, M. (2001). Is the male marriage premium due to selection? The effect of shotgun weddings on the return to marriage. *Journal of Population Economics, 14,* 313–328; Gupta, N. D., Smith, N., & Stratton, L. S. (2005, May). *Is marriage poisonous? Are relationships taxing? An analysis of the male marital wage differential in Denmark* (IZA DP No. 1591).

45. Bassuk, S. S., Glass, T. A., & Berkman, L. F. (1999). Social disengagement and incident cognitive decline in community-dwelling elderly persons. *Annals of Internal Medicine, 131,* 165–173; Byrne, G. J. A., & Raphael, B. (1997). The psychological symptoms of conjugal bereavement in elderly men over the first 13 months. *International Journal of Geriatric Psychiatry, 12,* 241–251.

46. Avlund, K., Damsgaard, M. T., & Holstein, B. E. (1998). Social relations and mortality. An eleven year follow-up study of 70-year-old men and women in Denmark. *Social Science & Medicine, 47,* 635–643; Bennett, K. M. (2002). Low level social engagement as a precursor of mortality among people in later life. *Age and Ageing, 31,* 165–168; Eng, P. M., Rimm, E. B., Fitzmaurice, G., & Kawachi, I. (2002). Social ties and change in social ties in relation to subsequent total and cause-specific mortality and coronary heart disease incidence in men. *Ameri-*

can *Journal of Epidemiology, 155*, 700–709; Cockerham, W. C., Hattori, H., & Yamori, Y. (2000). The social gradient in life expectancy: The contrary case of Okinawa in Japan. *Social Science & Medicine, 51*, 115–122; Shye, D., Mullooly, J. P., Freeborn, D. K., & Pope, C. R. (1995). Gender differences in the relationship between social network support and mortality: A longitudinal study of an elderly cohort. *Social Science and Medicine, 41*, 935–947; Siegel, J. M., & Kuykendall, D. H. (1990). Loss, widowhood, and psychological distress among the elderly. *Journal of Consulting and Clinical Psychology, 58*, 519–524; Stroebe, M. S. (1994). The broken heart phenomenon: An examination of the mortality of bereavement. *Journal of Community & Applied Social Psychology, 4*, 47–61.

47. Kiecolt-Glaser, J. K., Fisher, L. D., Ogrocki, P., Stout, J. C., Speicher, C. E., & Glaser, R. (1987). Marital quality, marital disruption, and immune function. *Psychosomatic Medicine, 49*, 13–34.

48. Adams, R. G., & Blieszner, R. (1995). Aging well with friends and family. *American Behavioral Scientist, 39*(2), 209–224.

49. Malarkey, W. B., Kiecolt-Glaser, J. K., Pearl, D., & Glaser, R. (1994). Hostile behavior during marital conflict alters pituitary and adrenal hormones. *Psychosomatic Medicine, 56*, 41–51; Seeman, T. E., & McEwen, B. S. (1996). Impact of social environment characteristics on neuroendocrine regulation. *Psychosomatic Medicine, 58*, 459–471.

50. Taylor, S. E., & Repetti, R. L. (1997). Health Psychology: What is an unhealthy environment and how does it get under the skin? *Annual Review of Psychology, 48*, 411–447.

51. Esterling, B. A., Kiecolt-Glaser, J. K., & Glaser, R. (1996). Psychosocial modulation of cytokine-induced natural killer cell activity in older adults. *Psychosomatic Medicine, 58*, 264–272; Moen, P., Dempster-McClain, D., & Williams, R. M. (1992). Successful aging: A life-course perspective on women's multiple roles and health. *American Journal of Sociology, 97*(6), 1612–1638.

52. Seeman, T. (1996). Social ties and health: The benefits of social integration. *Annals of Epidemiology, 6*, 442–451; Uchino, B. N., Kiecolt-Glaser, J. K., & Cacioppo, J. T. (1992). Age-related changes in cardiovascular response as a function of a chronic stressor and social support. *Journal of Personality and Social Psychology, 63*, 839–846; Uchino, B. N., Cacioppo, J. T., & Kiecolt-Glaser, J. K. (1996). The relationship between social support and physiological processes: A review with emphasis on underlying mechanisms and implications for health. *Psychological Bulletin, 119*(3), 488–531.

53. Kiecolt-Glaser, J. K., Newton, T., Cacioppo, J. T., MacCallum, R. C., Glaser, R., & Malarkey, W. B. (1996). Marital conflict and endocrine function: Are men really more physiologically affected than women? *Journal of Consulting and Clinical Psychology, 64*(2), 324–332; Kiecolt-Glaser, J. K., Loving, T. J., Stowell, J. R., Malarkey, W. B., Lemeshow, S. Dickinson, S. L., et al. (2005). Hostile marital interactions, proinflammatory cytokine production, and would healing. *Archives of General Psychiatry, 62,* 1377–1384.

54. Cohen, S. (2004). Social relationships and health. *American Psychologist,* 59676–684; Rook, K. S. (1984). The negative side of social interaction: Impact on psychological well-being. *Journal of Personality and Social Psychology, 46*(5), 1097–1108; Seeman, T. (1996). Social ties and health: The benefits of social integration. *Annals of Epidemiology, 6,* 442–451.

55. Cacioppo, J. T., Hughes, M. E., Waite, L. J., Hawkley, L. C., & Thisted, R. A. (2006). Loneliness as a specific risk factor for depressive symptoms: Cross-sectional and longitudinal analyses. *Psychology and Aging, 21,* 140–151; Cacioppo, J. T., Uchino, B. N., & Berntson, G. G. (1994). Individual differences in the autonomic origins of heart rate reactivity: The psychometrics of respiratory sinus arrhythmia and preejection period. *Psychophysiology, 31,* 412–419; Calabrese, J. R., Kling, M. A., & Gold, P. W. (1987). Alterations in immunocompetence during stress, bereavement, and depression: Focus on neuroendocrine regulation. *American Journal of Psychiatry, 144,* 1123–1134; Friedmann, E., Thomas, S. A., Liu, F., Morton, P. G., Chapa, D., Gottlieb, S. S. (2006). Relationship of depression, anxiety, and social isolation to chronic heart failure outpatient mortality. *American Heart Journal, 152*(5), 940.e1–940.e8; Kiecolt-Glaser, J. K., Rickers, D., George, J., Messick, G., Speicher, C. E., Garner, W., et al. (1984). Urinary cortisol levels, cellular immunocompetency, and lonliness in psychiatric inpatients. *Psychosomatic Medicine, 46*(1), 15–23; Steptoe, A., Wardle, J., & Marmot, M. (2005). Positive affect and health-related neuroendocrine, cardiovascular, and inflammatory processes. *Proceedings of the National Academy of sciences, 102*(18), 6508–6512.

CHAPTER 13

1. Apple, D. (1956). The social structure of grandparenthood. *American Anthropologist, 58,* 656–663.

2. Kornhaber, A., & Woodward, K. L. (1981). *Grandparents/grandchildren: The vital connection.* Garden City, NY: Anchor Press/Doubleday; Allen, J. S., Bruss, J., & Damasio, H. (2005). The aging brain: The cognitive

reserve hypothesis and hominid evolution. *American Journal of Human Biology, 17,* 673–689.

3. Barranti, C. C. R. (1985). The grandparent / grandchild relationship: Family resource in an era of voluntary bonds. *Family Relations, 34,* 343–352; Oyserman, D., Radin, N., & Saltz, E. (1994). Predictors of nurturant parenting in teen mothers living in three generational families. *Child Psychiatry and Human Development, 24,* 215–230.

4. Cohen, G. D. (2005). *The mature mind: The positive power of the aging brain.* New York: Basic Books.

5. Cattell, M. G. (1989). Knowledge and social change in Samia, Western Kenya. *Journal of Cross-Cultural Gerontology, 4,* 225–244.

6. Richman, J. A., & Flaherty, J. A. (1986). Childhood relationships, adult coping resources and depression. *Social Science & Medicine, 7,* 709–716; Shaw, B. A., Krause, N., Chatters, L. M., Connell, C. M., & Ingersoll-Dayton, B. (2004). Emotional support from parents early in life, aging, and health. *Psychology and Aging, 19*(1), 4–12.

7. Barrows, P. (1999). Fathers in parent-infant psychotherapy. *Infant Mental Health Journal, 20,* 333–345.

8. Gunnar, M. R. (1992). Reactivity of the hypothalamic-pituitary-adrenocortical system to stressors in normal infants and children. *Pediatrics, 90*(Suppl. 3), 491–479; Gunnar, M. R. (1998). Quality of care and buffering of neuroendocrine stress reactions: Potential effects on the developing human brain. *Preventive Medicine, 27,* 208–211; Schneider, M. L. (1992). Prenatal stress exposure alters postnatal behavioral expression under conditions of novelty challenge in rhesus monkey infants. *Developmental Psychobiology, 25,* 529–540; Seckl, J. R. (2004). Prenatal glucocorticoids and long-term programming. *European Journal of Endocrinology, 151,* U49–U62.

9. Field, T., Diego, M., Hernandez-Reif, M., Schanberg, S., Kuhn, C., Yando, R., et al. (2003). Pregnancy anxiety and comorbid depression and anger: Effects on the fetus and neonate. *Depression and Anxiety, 17,* 140–151.

10. Gur, R. C., Erwin, R. J., Gur, R. E., Zwil, A. S., Heimberg, C., & Kraemer, H. C. (1992). Facial emotion discrimination: II. Behavioral findings in depression. *Psychiatry Research, 42,* 241–251; Mikhailova, E. S., Vladimirova, T. V., Iznak, A. F., Tsusulkovskaya, E. J., & Sushko, N. V. (1996). Abnormal recognition of facial expression of emotions in depressed patients with major depression disorder and schizotypal personality disorder. *Biological Psychiatry, 40,* 697–705; Rubinow, D. R., & Post, R. M. (1992). Impaired recognition of affect in facial expression in depressed patients. *Biological Psychiatry, 31,* 947–953; Zuckerman,

B., Bauchner, H., Parker, S., & Cabral, H. (1990). Maternal depressive symptoms during pregnancy, and newborn irritability. *Developmental and Behavioral Pediatrics, 11,* 190–194.

11. Tronick, E. Z., & Gianino, A. F., Jr. (1986). The transmission of maternal disturbance to the Infant. In E. Z. Tronick & T. Field (Eds.), *New directions for child development: Vol. 34. Maternal depression and infant disturbance* (pp. 5–11). San Francisco: Jossey-Bass.

12. Dawson, G., Panagiotides, H., Klinger, L.G., & Hill, D. (1992). The role of frontal lobe functioning in the development of self-regulatory behavior. *Brain and Cognition, 20,* 152–175; Jones, N. A., Field, T., & Davalos, M. (2000). Right frontal EEG asymmetry and lack of empathy in preschool children of depressed mothers. *Child Psychiatry and Human Development, 30,* 189–204.

13. Cohen, S., & Wills, T. A. (1985). Stress, social support, and the buffering hypothesis. *Psychological Bulletin, 98,* 310–357; McLennan, J. D., & Offord, D. R. (2002). Should postpartum depression be targeted to improve child mental health? *Journal of the American Academy of Child and Adolescent Psychiatry, 41,* 28–35.

14. Collins, N. L., Dunkel-Schetter, C. D., Lobel, M., & Scrimshaw, S. C. M. (1993). Social support in pregnancy: Psychosocial correlates of birth outcomes and postpartum depression. *Journal of Personality and Social Psychology, 65,* 1243–1258.

15. Aitken, S. C. (2000). Fathering and faltering: "Sorry, but you don't have the necessary accoutrements". *Environment and Planning, A, 32,* 581–598.

16. Berg, S. J., & Wynne-Edwards, K. E. (2001). Changes in testosterone, cortisol, and estradiol levels in men becoming fathers. *Mayo Clinic Proceedings, 76,* 582–592; Gray, P. B., Kahlenberg, S. M., Barrett, E. S., Lipson, S. F., & Ellison, P. T. (2002). Marriage and fatherhood are associated with lower testosterone in males. *Evolution and Human Behavior, 23,* 193–201; Storey, A. E., Walsh, C. J., Quinton, R. L., & Wynne-Edwards, K. E. (2000). Hormonal correlates of paternal responsiveness in new and expectant fathers. *Evolution and Human Behavior, 21,* 79–95.

17. Booth, A., & Edwards, J. N. (1980). Fathers: The invisible parent. *Sex Roles, 6,* 445–456; Risman, B. J., & Park, K. (1988). Just the two of us: Parent-child relationships in single-parent homes. *Journal of Marriage and the Family, 50,* 1049–1062.

18. Grossman, K., Grossman, K. E., Fremmer-Bombik, E., Kindler, H., Scheuerer-Englisch, H., & Zimmermann, P. (2002). The uniqueness of

the child-father attachment relationship: Fathers' sensitive and challenging play as a pivotal variable in a 16-year longitudinal study. *Social Development, 11*, 307–331.

19. Harris, K. M., & Morgan, S. P. (1991). Fathers, sons, and daughters: Differential paternal involvement in parenting. *Journal of Marriage and the Family, 53*, 531–544.

20. Belsky, J., & Rovine, M. J. (1988). Nonmaternal care in the first year of life and the security of infant-parent attachment. *Child Development, 59*, 157–167; Caldera, Y. M. (2004). Paternal involvement and infant-father attachment: A Q-Set study. *Fathering, 2*, 191–210.

21. Lewis, C., & Lamb, M. E. (2003). Fathers' influences on children's development: The evidence from two-parent families. *European Journal of Psychology of Education, XVIII*, 211–226; Verschueren, K., & Marcoen, A. (1999). Representation of self and socioemotional competence in kindergarteners: Differential and combined effects of attachment to mother and to father. *Child Development, 70*, 183–201.

22. Lamb, M. E. (Ed.). (1997). *The role of the father in child development* (3rd ed.). New York: John Wiley & Sons; Lamb, M. E., & Lamb, J. E. (1976). The nature and importance of the father-infant relationship. *The Family Coordinator, 25*, 379–385.

23. Gottman, J. M., Katz, L. F., & Hooven, C. (1997). *Meta-emotion: How families communicate emotionally.* Hillsdale, NJ: Erlbaum; Harris, K. M., Furstenberg, F. F., Jr., & Marmer, J. K. (1998). Paternal involvement with adolescents in intact families: The influence of fathers over the life course. *Demography, 35*(2), 201–216; Ricks, S. S. (1985). Father-infant interactions: A review of empirical research. *Family Relations, 34*, 505–511; Rosenberg, J., & Wilcox, W. B. (2006). *The importance of fathers in the healthy development of children.* Washington, DC: U. S. Department of Health and Human Services, Administration for Children and Families, Administration on Children, Youth and Families, Children's Bureau, Office on Child Abuse and Neglect.

24. Amato, P. R., & Rivera, F. (1999). Paternal involvement and children's behavior problems. *Journal of Marriage and the Family, 61*, 375–384.

25. Dubowitz, H., Black, M. M., Cox, C. E., Kerr, M. A., Litrownik, A. J., Radhakrishna, A., et al. (2001). Father involvement and children's functioning at age 6 years: A multisite study. *Child Maltreatment, 6*(4), 300–309; White, L., & Gilbreth, J. G. (2001). When children have two fathers: Effects of relationships with stepfathers and noncustodial fathers on adolescent outcomes. *Journal of Marriage and Family, 63*, 155–167.

26. Volling, B. L., & Belsky, J. (1992). The contribution of mother-child and father-child relationships to the quality of sibling interaction: A longitudinal study. *Child Development, 63*, 1209–1222.
27. Amato, P. R., & Rezac, S. J. (1994). Contact with nonresident parents, interparental conflict, and children's behavior. *Journal of Family Issues, 15*(2), 191–207; Cabrera, N. J., Tamis-LeMonda, C. S., Bradley, R. H., Hofferth, S., & Lamb, M. E. (2000). Fatherhood in the twenty-first century. *Child Development, 71*(1), 127–136.
28. Mahoney, D., & Restak, R. (1998). *The longevity strategy: How to live to 100 using the brain-body connection.* New York: John Wiley and Sons.

CHAPTER 14

1. Frank, A. W. (2000). The standpoint of storyteller. *Qualitative Health Research, 10*(3), 354–365.
2. Mahoney, D., & Restak, R. (1998). *The longevity strategy: How to live to 100 using the brain-body connection.* New York: John Wiley and Sons.
3. Caldwell, R. (2005). At the confluence of memory and meaning – life review with older adults and families: using narrative therapy and the experessive arts to re-member and re-author stories of resilience. *The Family Journal: Counseling and Therapy for Couples and Families, 13,* 172–175.
4. Hanaoka, H., & Okamura, H. (2004). Study on effects of life review activities on the quality of life of the elderly: a randomized trial. *Psychotherapy and Psychosomatics, 73,* 302–311.
5. Haber, D. (2006). Life review: implementation, theory, research, and therapy. *International Journal of Aging and Human Development, 63*(2), 153–171.
6. Greene, R. R. (1986). Social work with the aged and their families. New York: Aldine De Gruyter; Sherman, E., & Peak, T. (1991). Patterns of reminiscence and the assessment of late life adjustment. *Journal of Gerontological Social Work. 161*(1-2), 59–74.
7. Maercker, A., & Zollner, T. (2002). Life review therapie als spezifische form der behandlung posttraumatischer belastungsstorungen im alter. *Verhaltensth & Verhaltensmed, 23,* 120–140; McInnis-Dittrich, K. (1996). Adapting life-review for elderly female survivors of childhood sexual abuse. *Families in society: the Journal of Contemporary Human Services, 77*(3), 166–173.
8. Maercker, A. (2002). Life-review technique in the treatment of PTSD in elderly patients: Rationale and three single case studies. *Journal of Clinical Geropsychology, 8,* 239–249.

9. Sherman, E. (1991). Reminiscentia: cherished objects as memorabilia in late-life reminiscence. *International Journal of Aging and Human Development, 33*(2), 89– 100.

10. Haight, B. K., Michel, Y., & Hendrix, S. (2000). The extended effects of the life review in nursing home residents. *International Journal of Aging and Human Development, 63*(2), 153– 171.

11. Hausman, C.P. (1980). Life Review Therapy. *Journal of Gerontological Social Work, 3*(2), 31–37.

12. McInnis-Dittrich, K. (1996). Adapting life-review for elderly female survivors of childhood sexual abuse. *Families in society: the Journal of Contemporary Human Services, 77*(3), 166–173.

13. Brooks, B. M., Mcneil, J. E., Rose, F. D., Attree, E. A., leadbetter, A. G. (1999). Route learning in a case of amnesia: a preliminary investigation into the efficacy of training in a virtual environment. *Neuropsychological Rehabilitation, 9*(1), 63–76(14); Cavallini, E., Pagnin, A., Vecchi, T. (2003). Aging and everyday memory: the beneficial effect of memory training. *Archives of Gerontology and Geriatrics, 37,* 241 – 257; Floyd, M., & Scogin, F. (1997). Effects of memory training on the subjective memory functioning and mental health of older adults: a meta-analysis. *Psychology and Aging, 12*(1), 150–161; Madden, D. J., Turkington, T. G., Provenzale, J. M., Denny, L. L., Hawk, T. C., Gottlob, L. R., et al. (1999). Adult age differences in the functional neuroanatomy of verbal recognition memory. *Human Brain Mapping, 7,* 115–135; Rapp, S., Brenes, G., & Marsh, A. P. (2002). Memory enhancement training for older adults with mild cognitive impairment: a preliminary study. *Aginig and Mental Health, 6*(1), 5–11; Schaie, K. W., & Willis, S. L. (1986). Can decline in adult intellectual functioning be reversed? *Developmental Psychology, 22,* 223–232; Thompson, G. (2005). Cognitive-training programs for older adults: What are they and can they enhance mental fitness? *Educational Gerontology, 31,* 603–626.

14. Rand-Giovannetti, E., Chua, E. F., Driscoll, A. E., Schacter, D. L., Albert, M. S., & Sperling, R. A. (2006). Hippocampal and neocortical activation during repetitive encoding in older persons. *Neurobiology of Aging, 27,* 173–182; Valenzuela, M. J., Jones, M., Wen, W., Rae, C., Graham, S., Shnier, R., Sachdev, P. (2003). Memory training alters hippocampal neurochemistry in healthy elderly. *Neuroreport, 14*(10), 1333–1337.

15. Neely, A. S., & Backman, L. (1995). Effects of multifactorial memory training in old age: generalized across tasks and individuals. *The Journals of Gerontology, 50*(3), P134–P140; Rapp, S., Brenes, G., & Marsh,

A. P. (2002). Memory enhancement training for older adults with mild cognitive impairment: a preliminary study. *Aginig and Mental Health*, 6(1), 5–11.

16. Flynn, T. M., & Storandt, M. (1990). Supplemental group discussions in memory training for older adults. *Psychology and Aging*, 5(2), 178–181; Mohs, R. C., Ashman, T. A., Jantzen, K., Albert, M., Brandt, J., Gordon, B., et al. (1998). A study of the efficacy of a comprehensive memory enhancement program in healthy elderly persons. *Psychiatry Research*, 77(3), 183–195; Rapp, S., Brenes, G., & Marsh, A. P. (2002). Memory enhancement training for older adults with mild cognitive impairment: a preliminary study. *Aginig and Mental Health*, 6(1), 5–11; Troyer, A. K., (2001). Improving memory knowledge, satisfaction, and functioning, via an education and intervention program for older adults. *Neuropsychology, Development and Cogntion*, 8(4), 256–268.

17. Noice, H., Noice, T., Perrig-Chiello, P., Perrig, W. (1999). Improving memory in older adults by instructing them in professional actors' learning strategies. *Applied Cognitive Psychology*, 13(4), 315–328.

18. Oswald, W. D., Gunzelmann, T., Rupperecht, R., & Hagen, B. (2006). Differential effects of single versus combined cognitive and physical training with older adults: The simA study in a 5-year perspective. *European Journal of Ageing*, 3, 179–192; Rebok, G. W., & Plude, D. J. (2001). Relation of physical activity to memory functioning in older adults: the memory workout program. *Educational Gerontology*, 27(3-4), 241–259.

19. Noice, H., Noice, T., Perrig-Chiello, P., Perrig, W. (1999). Improving memory in older adults by instructing them in professional actors' learning strategies. *Applied Cognitive Psychology*, 13(4), 315–328.

20. Luks, A. (1988, October). Helper's high. *Psychology Today*, 22(10), 34–42.

21. Field, T. M., Hernandez-Reif, M., Quintino, O., Schanberg, S., & Kuhn, C. (1998). Elder retired volunteers benefit from giving massage therapy to infants. *The Journal of Applied Gerontology*, 17(2), 229–239.

22. McClelland, D., McClelland, D. C., & Kirchnit, C. (1988). The effect of motivational arousal through films on salivary immunoglobulin A. *Psychology and Health*, 2, 31–52.

23. U.S. Census Bureau (2002). *Statistical Abstract of the United States: 2002*. United States Summary Washington, DC, 2004

24. Midlarsky, E., & Kahana, E. (1994). *Altruism in later life*. Thousand Oaks, CA: Sage Publications.

25. Dulin, P. L. & Hill, R. D. (2003). Relationships between altruistic activity and positive and negative affect among low-income older adult ser-

vice providers. *Aging & Mental Health*, 7(4), 294–299; Greenfield, E. A., & Marks, N. F. (2004). Formal volunteering as a protective factor for older adults' psychological well-being. *The Journals of Gerontology*, 59B(5), S258– S264; Hunter, K. I., & Linn, M. W. (1980–1981). Psychosocial differencesbetween elderly volunteers and non-volunteers. *International Journal of Aging and Human Development*, 12, 205–213; Morrow-Howell, N., Hinterlong, J., Rozario, P. A., & Tang, F. (2003). Effects of volunteering on the well-being of older adults. *Journal of Gerontology: Social Sciences*, 58B(3), S137–S145; Musick, M. A., & Wilson, J. (2003). Volunteering and depression: The role of psychological and social resources in different age groups. *Social Science & Medicine*, 56, 259–269; Schwartz, C., Meisenhelder, J. B., Ma, Y., & Reed, G. (2003). Altruistic social interest behaviors are associated with better mental health. *Psychosomatic Medicine*, 65, 778–785.

26. Brown, J. W., & Braver, T. S. (2005). Learned predictions of error likelihood in the anterior cingulate cortex. *Science*, 307, 1118-1121; Brown, J., Cooper-Kuhn, C. M., Kempermann, G., van Praag, H., Winkler, J., Gage, F. H., & Kuhn, H. G. (2003). Enriched environment and physical activity stimulate hippocampal but not olfactory bulb neurogenesis. *European Journal of Neuroscience*, 17, 2042–2046; Musick, M. A., Herzog, A. R., & House, J. S. (1999). Volunteering and mortality among older adults: Findings from a national sample. *The Journals of Gerontology*. 54B(3), S173–S180; Oman, D., Thoresen, C. E., & McMahon, K. (1999). Volunteerism and mortality among the community-dwelling elderly. *Journal of Health Psychology*, 4(3), 1359–1053.

27. Brown, J. W., & Braver, T. S. (2005). Learned predictions of error likelihood in the anterior cingulate cortex. *Science*, 307, 1118-1121; Brown, J., Cooper-Kuhn, C. M., Kempermann, G., van Praag, H., Winkler, J., Gage, F. H., & Kuhn, H. G. (2003). Enriched environment and physical activity stimulate hippocampal but not olfactory bulb neurogenesis. *European Journal of Neuroscience*, 17, 2042–2046.

28. Vaillant, G. E. (2002). *Aging well*. New York, NY: Little, Brown and Company.

29. Levy, B. R. (1996). Improving memory in old age by implicit self-stereotyping. *Journal of Personality and Social Psychology*, 71, 1092–1107; Levy, B. R., Slade, M. D., & Kasl, S. V. (2002). Longitudinal benefit of positive self-perceptions of aging on functional health. *Journal of Gerontology*, 57B(5), 409– 417.

INDEX

Note: Italicized page locators refer to illustrations; tables are noted with *t*.

initiative *vs.* guilt, in Erikson's
  model, 133*t*
inner world, agelessness of, 176
insecure attachment
  brain development and, 43
  children, stress, and, 42
insight, sleep and development of,
  203–4
insular cortex, function of, 46
integrity
  despair *vs.*, in Erikson's model,
    133*t*
  in Vaillant's reformulation of
    Erikson's stages, 135*t*
interdependence, challenge of, 21
intergenerational relationships
  alterations in, 23–25
  appreciating need for connected-
    ness in, 55
internal feelings, social judgments
  and, 162
internal world, reflection and, 169
interpersonal neurobiology, life of
  social brain and, 36
intimacy
  healthy brain and, 38
  isolation *vs.*, in Erikson's model,
    133*t*
  in Vaillant's reformulation of
    Erikson's stages, 135*t*
Iroquois, three sisters creation
  myth of, 30
isolation
  brain and impact of, 99–100
  countering, ideas for, 261–62
  diminished well-being and, 222
  factors contributing to, 221
  intimacy *vs.*, in Erikson's model,
    133*t*
  sleep disturbances and, 204

James, W., 166, 180, 188
Jessel, G., 142
Jesus Christ, 126, 152, 249
job challenges, cognitive reserves
  and, 81, 82
job sharing, intergenerational, 261
Jung, C., 43

Kahn, R. L., 209
keeper of the meaning, in Vaillant's reformulation of Erikson's stages, 135*t*
Keller, H., 29
King, M. L., Jr., 57–59, 126, 127,
  152
Kipling, R., 21
knee-jerk reflex, 160
knowledge
  leaping to wisdom from, 121–22
  stories and transmission of, 250
  see also learning; wisdom

language
  brain and gender differences in,
    109
  development of, 90
  failing senses and, 210
  in late adulthood, 179–80
  left cerebral hemisphere and,
    104, 186
Lao Tzu, 217
lateral specialization
  evolution of social brain and,
    102
  in young adulthood, 94
laughter, benefits of, 215–17
learning
  caloric restriction and, 198–99
  estrogen receptors and, 111
  exercise and, 202